Medical School Admissions:
The Insider's Guide

Medical School Admissions:
The Insider's Guide

John A. Zebala
&
Daniel B. Jones

Revised & updated by
Stephanie B. Jones

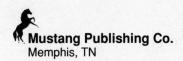

Mustang Publishing Co.
Memphis, TN

Copyright © 1989, 1992 by John A. Zebala, Daniel B. Jones, and
Stephanie B. Jones.

All rights reserved, including the right of reproduction in whole or
in part in any form. Published in the United States of America by
Mustang Publishing Co., Inc., P.O. Box 3004, Memphis, TN 38173.
Manufactured and printed in the U.S.A.

Distributed to the trade in the USA by National Book Network, Lan-
ham, Maryland.

Library of Congress Cataloging in Publication Data
Zebala, John A.
     Medical school admissions: the insider's guide / John A.
Zebala, Daniel B. Jones. -- Rev. & updated by Stephanie B. Jones.
        p. cm.
     ISBN 0-914457-49-7 : $10.95
     1. Medical colleges--United States--Admission. 2. Medical
colleges--United States--Entrance requirements.   I. Jones,
Daniel B.   II. Jones, Stephanie B.   III. Title.
R838.4.Z42   1992
610' .71' 173--dc20   92-50414
                                                       CIP

Printed on acid-free paper. ∞

10 9 8 7 6 5 4 3 2

Wherever the art
of medicine is loved,
there also is love of humanity.

Hippocrates

Acknowledgments

This book is dedicated to Keith Bernstein, Doug Lytle, Steve Taylor, Brian Wong, Francis Barany, Mary Burton, Carol Snow, Alfonso Torres, Jane Crawford, and Amy Burnham—undergraduate and graduate friends without whose knowledge, inspiration, and sometimes irritation this book would have never been written.

We would also like to thank the many Deans of Admission who gave thoughtful commentary on this book.

Special thanks also to the students accepted at Cornell University Medical College, Johns Hopkins, Yale, Harvard, UCLA, University of Pennsylvania, Columbia, Washington University, and New York University who contributed their successful AMCAS essays. These students include (but are not limited to) Wendell Danforth, John Linsalata, Matt Pease, Jeff Budoff, Hal Baker, Dan Medalie, Karl Illig, Daniel Javit, Fred Lee, Perry Sutaria, and Marcia Simpson.

Most importantly, we would like to thank our parents, who supported us throughout the admissions process not too long ago.

John A. Zebala
Daniel B. Jones
Stephanie B. Jones

Foreword

At present, over 30,000 individuals apply for the 17,000 positions available yearly at the 127 medical schools in the United States. Both applicants and schools take the annual application process most seriously and expend a great deal of time and effort making it work favorably for them.

To insure consistency and continuity, most medical school admissions committee members serve more than one annual processing cycle. In contrast, students attempt to navigate the course from applicant to matriculant only once. Therefore, it's most reasonable for them to ask at the beginning, "What can I do to help my chances of being selected by the school of my choice?"

In what follows, John Zebala and Daniel Jones, two successful applicants to Cornell University Medical College, offer their firsthand account of "what works." For those who endured the admissions process several decades ago, it is an eye-opening account of the present. For those seeking to start the path towards a medical education, it is a thought-provoking collection of organized steps and considerations for your assistance.

In practice, the medical school admissions process initially reduces you, the individual, to several sets of numbers (GPAs and MCAT scores), lists of courses and accomplishments, an essay, and several letters of recommendation. In short, it makes you create a paper caricature of yourself. Next, admissions committees review thousands of such "paper individuals" to select a group of manageable size to interview. Finally, from the hundreds interviewed, a few individuals are admitted to fill classes of 90 to 170.

How do you survive this process and effectively represent yourself? John and Daniel offer here their thoughts on doing just that. Is everything they suggest suitable for everyone? Of course not. But you should consider their suggestions and decide which are suitable for you. It's certainly helpful and worth your time.

Remember, medical school admissions committees are seeking intelligent, thoughtful, caring, motivated individuals to fill their classes. To be successful, you must demonstrate those qualities which suit you for entering the medical profession, as well as those which make you a unique, interesting individual.

My advice: Be yourself, and don't let the real you get lost in the process.

Gordon F. Fairclough, Jr., Ph.D.
Dean of Admissions
Cornell University Medical College

Contents

Introduction

The best effect of any book is that it excites the reader to self activity. Thomas Carlyle

Treat people as if they were what they ought to be, and you help them to become what they are capable of being.
Johann W. von Goethe

One of the most difficult things to do when applying to medical school is deciphering which advice is accurate and which is not. The main problem is that most of the people giving advice have never actually gone through the admissions process themselves. That's why this book is unique.

As medical students, our firsthand knowledge of the admissions process will probably be the best and most realistic advice you'll ever hear. Often, books and counselors do more to *dis*courage the applicant than *en*courage. Well, we're not going to tell you that in order to be a doctor you have to make straight A's, climb Mount Everest, or be Ms. Wonderful-Everything, because the fact is, you don't.

We believe that getting into medical school is not an insurmountable task, and that what most doctors actually do in their everyday practice does not require a genius intellect or qualify them for a Nobel Prize. Instead, we believe that the whole admissions process is a formula, a game with set rules. If you play the game by the rules, you'll get in. It's that simple. Our goal is to tell you exactly what the formula entails, as we have learned from our own experience and from interviews with admissions committee members.

A major attraction in our book, we believe, is the large number of actual AMCAS essays (a.k.a. "personal statements") collected from students admitted to top medical colleges around the country. Applicants spend months writing and perfecting their essays, and every year premedical students scramble and search for successful essays to read. We think the collection will be invaluable in showing you how broad the range of potential topics is, and it should give you an idea of what gets admissions committees excited. Plus, we hope the essays will inspire your own creativity and relieve some anxiety.

Another extremely anxious time for the applicant to medical school is the interview. The uncertainties and fears surrounding this part of the process can be a nightmare. So, we have accumulated a list of questions that interviewers have asked applicants during actual interviews. We have also researched what interviewers typically seek during an interview. Applicants rarely know how their application and responses are evaluated, or what questions are likely to arise in the interview. These pieces of information are exactly what you need to turn what might be just good interviews into really great interviews.

We also recommend additional reading, rank the country's medical schools, provide the latest information on the MCAT, and include a timetable that allows you to track and check your progress throughout the application process.

Most importantly, we encourage premedical students to apply with confidence, and we suggest ways they can properly market their strengths.

It may also be useful to mention what this book is **not**. This book will not help you decide if medicine is for you. That decision can come only from working in a hospital and by observing physicians. Likewise, we make no attempt to glorify medicine; we'll leave that to *Saint Elsewhere* and *M*A*S*H*. Instead, we hope to convince you that half the battle in the medical school admissions game is thinking positively and knowing how to work within the system.

Once you have these insights, you'll realize that it's not necessary to be cutthroat to get into medical school. On the contrary, the best physicians are not chemistry lab nerds who would sabotage a neighbor's experiment. They are thoughtful, caring, well-rounded people with wide-ranging interests. If you would like to be this kind of physician, read on, because what follows is the ultimate set of inside tips for medical school admissions success!

Chapter 1

Premedical Preparation

Basically, there are three types of premedical students:

The first is the most familiar. They knew they were going to be physicians from the very beginning. At age two they were playing with a stethoscope. In high school, they chose a college based on how it would affect their medical school acceptance. The second, and probably largest, group are those who decide to undertake the quest for medical school in their undergraduate years. The third group consists of people who decided on medical school after college graduation—and sometimes after being established in another career.

While different in many ways, all three groups share two common misconceptions. First, they think that just because medicine draws upon science, every premed should major in biology or chemistry. Second, they think the quality of their college and their major are deciding factors in their admission to medical school.

In fact, nothing could be further from the truth. Because the spectrum of physicians is so broad, there is no preferred major to enter the medical profession. In some cases, the quality of the undergraduate university can affect your chances of admission to medical school, but usually it is irrelevant. (An important exception are undergraduate colleges that have an affiliated medical school. More on this later.)

Let's be honest. Except for some professional sports, medicine is the highest paying profession in the United States today, so it's not too surprising that so many "willing and dedicated" people are anxious to secure one of the limited spaces in medical schools. Further, it's also not surprising that many premedical students are conscious (almost paranoid) about the most minor details of their undergraduate curriculum. The unfortunate reality is that the paranoia is unfounded. It's based on pervasive myths spread by other premedical students, not on the true details that admissions committees consider important.

So what *is* important? At the risk of over-simplifying, you must have (or create) a quality that makes you stand out from the pack. Standing out is another way of saying that you are "interesting," and "interesting" is what medical schools go for.

Once you decide to pursue medical school, it's essential that you remain you. It's okay (indeed, we heartily recommend it) to explore your talents and curiosity in college. Go ahead and learn to scuba dive or take a course on Emily Dickinson, if that's what you'd like to do. With this philosophy, you need not worry about the person next to you all the time, and you'll be much more relaxed. If you want to become a "doctor to the stars" in Hollywood, get a degree in business or, better yet, cinema. Don't laugh! Patients want to be able to relate to their doctors.

If you are like most premedical students, you probably don't know what kind of doctor you want to become. So our advice is simple: major in whatever interests you.

Planning Your Undergraduate Study

In the long run of history, the censor and the inquisitor have always lost. The only sure weapon against bad ideas is better ideas. The source of better ideas is wisdom. The surest path to wisdom is a liberal education. A. Whitney Griswold

When medical schools receive an applicant's grades, they look at the overall grade point average, as well as the GPA derived exclusively from science courses.

Now, you non-science majors probably realize your potential disadvantage in this procedure. That is, if an English major gets a C in freshman chemistry, he'll have a pitiful science grade point average, because he won't have many science courses to average with the C. That lone C will stand as indicative of mediocre scientific ability—though it may in fact be a false representation.

We know all the sob stories about your bad semester that year. You had family problems, girl- or boyfriend problems, a lingering case of beriberi, etc. Unfortunately, these stories are often true and relevant, but medical schools give little if any consideration to such deficiencies unless you show marked improvement and progress later in your transcript.

So if you're a non-science major and you've got a poor science grade, you'll need to spend extra effort to raise your science average. If your grade is poor in a course, take the course again if you can get the bad grade erased. If you can't get it erased but merely averaged with the new grade, we don't advise taking the course over. Instead, take a more advanced science course, which will average the low grade plus look better and more purposeful on your transcript.

Medical schools today seem to have had enough of the eggheads, and they are leaning more towards people with degrees in the liberal arts and science majors who are "well-rounded." In fact, economics majors have some of the highest percentages of acceptance to medical colleges, and biology majors among the lowest, within each of their respective groups. (Of course, this doesn't mean you should switch your major to economics, because an alternative interpretation of this statistic is possible. That is, a higher percentage of mediocre applicants are biology majors, since nearly every biology major applies to med school.)

We have a friend, a straight-A biomedical engineer, who interviewed at Washington University. One of the first things they told him was, "Frankly, Mr. Smith, we've found that English majors make the best doctors." Don't get us wrong—he had no trouble getting accepted there. The point is, it's wrong to think that you must be a science major to be a doctor, or that being a science major will give you an advantage when applying to medical school.

A premedical student must fulfill certain science requirements: one year of inorganic chemistry, one year of organic chemistry, one year of physics, and one year of biology. Other required subjects, such as English and calculus, vary with different med schools. Past these, you can major in almost anything.

At many schools, the science courses are extremely difficult, especially at schools with a good science reputation. This is also often the case at large universities, where classes with over 700 premedical students are common. Usually, organic chemistry is the "weed-out" class. Well, here's some good news: you don't need to be part of a "weed-out," and you don't have to sit back and take it. If you can take organic elsewhere, where it's easier and maybe even cheaper, then by all means do so. An A is an A on your transcript, no matter where you got it.

All of you have heard people say that they were going to take so-and-so science course because they thought it would help them in medical school or look good to admissions committees. This is the most absurd way of assuring yourself an A or an honors later in medical school. Medical schools apparently agree with us, since they strongly discourage students from taking courses that resemble the first year's curriculum in med school.

The best way to get an A in med school is simply to work hard for it when the time comes. Unless you are truly interested in the sciences, you will not make your transcript look more impressive by taking med school-level courses as an undergraduate. In fact, you'll probably make it look worse, because your grade point average could be lower. Anyway, when you don't have to worry about advanced courses, you'll have more time to go to the beach or the mountains.

The hardest hurdle to jump is getting into a medical school. Therefore, any method that lets you take short cuts, have fun, and still get in is a perfectly acceptable alternative to killing yourself by studying 24 hours a day for courses that you may never use again in your life.

The rationale is simple: you'll learn everything you need to know to become a doctor in medical school. You don't need to be Isaac Newton's clone, and you don't need advanced courses on the undergraduate level (biochemistry sometimes being the exception). You simply must show aptitude and a minimum amount of knowledge about science so you can survive the medical curriculum.

Completing your undergraduate degree with good grades merely tells a medical college you have the *stamina* to persevere for four years, and do it well. In general, it's a good indication of your ability to do well in medical school, because the coursework in med school is just like undergraduate coursework, but at much higher endurance levels.

Picking the Right Undergraduate College

It is all one to me if a man comes from Sing Sing or Harvard. We hire a man, not his history. Henry Ford

Many medical schools will tell applicants from junior colleges and some state universities that, statistically, they are at a distinct disadvantage to applicants who went to a private university or a respected state school. The reason is that GPAs earned at the former are not deemed as valuable as those from more competitive schools. We agree that this is unfair, especially since many people must attend such schools for economic or geographic reasons.

So what do you do if you go to Mediocre State Tech? Pack it up and transfer? Certainly not! You'll just have to be that much better than others, and your GPA should be that much higher.

Does this mean that med schools make numerical adjustments on GPAs depending on what college you attended? Yes, many do. Obviously, this hurts individuals high on the scale whose grades are adjusted down, since it's impossible to achieve higher than a 4.0 average. On the other hand, admissions committees often inflate the value of grades from prestigious colleges, so a lot of boneheads get in from top schools. Hey, who said life is fair?

You basically have two choices: transfer to a better school, if that's the problem, or work really hard where you are. We favor doing the latter, rather than worrying about the alma mater.

However, there is one case when we suggest you transfer. If you have the choice, always go to a university with a medical school. Twenty percent of the students at some medical schools attended that school as an undergraduate. Obviously, the university has to show that it believes in its own product, so, statistically, its own premeds have a notable advantage over other applicants when they apply to their university's med school.

Nevertheless, if you are good, it doesn't matter where you went to college. You'll stand out sooner or later. Besides, medical colleges have devised a way out of such subjective dilemmas—it's called the MCAT. It turns all students—whether they're from Yale or Arkansas Tech—into a cold, objective number. If you do well on the MCAT, you'll get into medical school.

So don't lose sleep about which undergraduate school you should attend. Go to the college that appeals to you because of location, price, curriculum, sports program, or other personal reasons. If chemistry and physics are your thing, then go to a school known for sciences. The same logic applies if you're interested in drama or art.

The real bottom line is how you measure up as a person. College may give you the only opportunity to enjoy and explore things that really excite you other than medicine. After all, health professionals treat people and must be people themselves, not simply mechanics fixing machines. They must have a well-rounded intelligence as well as scientific knowledge, since they deal with incredible technology—and everyday patients.

So don't be one-dimensional, the stereotypical premed nerd, grinding away for hours in the library and the lab. Use your undergraduate experience creatively and explore college opportunities to their fullest. It will do wonders to shape you as a whole person, and it will make you a much better doctor someday.

Chapter 2

Power Techniques
for Higher Grades

It's common knowledge that good grades are essential in gaining acceptance to medical school. The problem is, "good" is usually not explicitly defined.

For those who don't have perfect grade point averages, believing the philosophy of "the higher the GPA, the better" can cause some real mental anguish—especially if you use the class valedictorian as your standard. On the other hand, you're kidding yourself if you think medical schools admit students at the bottom of their class. Of course, reality is somewhere between these two extremes.

Here's a real life example: During our volunteer work in an urban emergency room, a physician told us he had a 2.0 average as an undergraduate majoring in chemistry. After graduation, he didn't know what he wanted to do with his life, so he went to Africa with the Peace Corps for two years. Helping a lot of suffering people there convinced him that medicine was his calling. He returned to the United States and took a year of graduate courses, after which he entered medical school.

In contrast, we know an applicant from a prestigious college who had nearly perfect grades and MCAT scores. Almost every medical school rejected him. The problem was that nothing in his record made him unique or revealed a *sincere desire* to study medicine.

The lesson, then, is simple: there's not always a clear grade break determining who will and who won't be accepted. In fact, some medical schools don't even have a minimum GPA requirement. For the sake of being realistic though, you should have at least a 3.0—unless your MCAT scores are quite high or you have truly special circumstances in your personal life.

Some of you may think such grades are difficult to attain. However, we believe a 3.0 or higher is a realistic goal for just about anybody, if you go about it correctly.

Techniques for Grade Point Success

Although you may be familiar with some of the techniques outlined in this chapter, many people do not adhere to even the most basic points. The irony is, those who don't practice good study habits are often the same students who complain about how difficult their courses are. Therefore, if you fall into this group, or even if you don't, refresh your memory about good, basic study techniques. These concepts can make your courses seem much easier.

1. Obtain old exams.

The first golden rule to success in college courses is to study old exams. Professors are not so creative that they can devise completely original exam questions each year. In fact, they often don't have time to change the test much at all. So you'll frequently see either the same questions, or questions that are very similar, to those on old exams.

Some of you may think, "I don't need old exams, because if I really know the material I'll ace the exam anyway." We thought the same thing until reality (and a few C's) hit us in the face. Many questions that involve concepts require insight from the student, and insight requires time—usually more than allowed on exams. Exposure to similar or identical concepts days before an exam will put you way ahead of others who are seeing the problem for the first time.

Using this technique, a two-letter increase in your grades is common (i.e., from a C to an A). You can probably get old exams from upper classmates, teaching assistants, or sometimes the professor, if you explain that the majority of the class has them. Hustling for old exams is a skill you should learn and constantly refine, since you'll need it later in medical school, where exams are even more repetitive and predictable.

Of course, this must all be in the realm of honest, ethical behavior. Cheaters do not get into med school.

2. Take a reasonable course load.

Another golden rule to success in college: don't overload your class schedule. Most students realize that if they had more time, they could do better in their courses. In other words, the problem is not that certain courses are intrinsically difficult; it's that they are time consuming, and they take time away from all your other courses.

Don't get the wrong idea—we are not suggesting that you attend school part-time. Rather, we suggest you eliminate super-macho schedules. For example, some students think they can take four laboratory courses in one semester and still get a 3.7 GPA. If you can, more power to you, and we'll congratulate you when you get the Nobel Prize. However, most students get only poor grades and lots of stress.

A reasonable schedule means more time. More time means less stress. Less stress means you will enjoy the courses you're taking and think more deeply about them. It's ironic that, although a university exists to foster creative thinking, most students feel such time pressure that creative thought becomes impossible.

3. Study alone.

For the most part, we advise you to study alone.

Many people insist that group study is best because you're forced to think hard about the topic when you must explain it to someone else. As a result, they say, group study will expose weaknesses in your comprehension of a subject.

It sounds good, but most group study doesn't work out that way. Instead of quizzing each other and discussing topics relevant to the course, you spend your time gossiping about the party last weekend. If your study partner is attractive, you won't be concentrating on the material. Plus, there's usually somebody in the group who only wants to be tutored, and he's so far behind that he can't contribute anything. (He's usually the same person who asks you for lecture notes because he felt class wasn't as important as his sleep.)

Don't misunderstand—sometimes it is appropriate to form a group to tackle class material. If a professor is disorganized and confusing, a study session with good students can clear up tough concepts. And topics which require a lot of memorization are easier to learn if another person quizzes you (e.g. organic chemistry reactions).

But nine times out of ten, you're better off studying alone, without all the distractions of a group.

4. Choose the proper study environment.

Study in a quiet place that's not too comfortable. Some people claim they can study on a couch while they watch *Monday Night Football*. For most students, however, this is the first step to disaster.

Courses like physics and chemistry require deep, sustained concentration, and distractions like TV and radio only hinder good studying. College life comes with many freedoms that can make grades suffer if a student can't impose self-discipline. Part of being a physician (or an adult, for that matter) is knowing when to work and when to play. Developing such habits early will make life much easier in the future.

A library-like environment is where you will study most efficiently. If you study on your bed, odds are you'll fall asleep. Unfortunately, many libraries are uncomfortable. You should find a place where you can think intensely for long hours.

5. Highlight your books.

Highlight and write in your textbooks. Students from public high schools, where it was a capital offense to put even a light pencil mark in a textbook, may have a tough time with this. However, universities require students to purchase their own books, and usually at high prices. Since you own these expensive texts, it's totally acceptable and certainly advisable to write in them.

Highlighting is a good way to filter out minor details, and it's an excellent way to review for exams. If you don't write in your texts because you want to keep them in pristine condition, you're making studying much more difficult than it need be. Besides, the resale value of marked-up books is exactly the same as clean books.

6. Make flash cards.

Most people do not like to use flash cards because it reminds them of learning multiplication tables in third grade. But flash cards are the most useful—and least used—study technique.

Flash cards appear to be expensive and time-consuming to make. This is true only if you wait until the end of a course to make them. We have found that folding a regular sheet of paper into sixteen squares and then cutting them out makes the best size (and least expensive) flash cards. Use paper clips to keep them in convenient bundles, and make them as you go along with your studies.

For instance, when you highlight a concept in a book, write it down on your flash card in the form of a question, with the question on one side and the answer on the other. Once you've made the cards, even learning material that involves simple regurgitation will be easier. Since you already wrote them, reviewing the material will be fast and as good, if not better, than being quizzed by another student.

7. Keep a social life.

Although many college students tend to socialize at the expense of good grades, some premeds go to the opposite extreme and withdraw entirely from the fun of college life. But that's a mistake, because social relaxation provides an excellent release for tension and prevents burnout. Moreover, a moderate social life will actually enhance your academics. You'll find that wasting a whole evening at the movies or at the local tavern will put you in a much better mood to study organic chemistry the next morning.

A social life will keep your eyes open to the rest of the world and will remind you that there's more to life than the basement of the library. Your undergraduate years should be some of the best years of your life, so it only makes sense to enjoy them as much as possible.

8. Understand concepts that seem unlikely to appear on the exam.

Professors realize there are certain topics with which most students have problems. Many times we would say to ourselves, "He'd never test us on this stuff. It's too hard, and he spent only five minutes discussing it." Guess what? The obscure stuff would always be on the exam, and they were always the questions that most of the class got wrong.

Exams are constructed with a bell curve in mind: there are questions everyone should be able to answer, questions some people should be able to answer, and a few questions only the top students will get. Topics that seem trivial and ambiguous are, as one professor told us, "excellent material with which to separate the A students from the B students."

Look at it this way: it's just a game, so be a smart player and pay attention to even the most minor details.

9. Don't memorize when you can understand.

If you can learn something by either memorizing it or conceptually understanding it, always choose the latter. Generally, it's less efficient to memorize many details than to understand a general principle from which you can derive the specifics.

Learning things this way will help you excel in courses like physics and chemistry, where exam questions are not identical to, but similar to, the homework problems. If you understand the principle well, you'll be able to apply the concept to the problem on the exam.

Improving Grades a Little Bit More: Being Assertive

Although studying hard is probably the single most important factor in achieving high grades, there are times when being aggressive may be just what it takes to push you from a B+ to an A-.

Unfortunately, some students take this philosophy to the extreme, and it only works against them. They are perceived as obnoxious, and teaching assistants and students avoid helping them. Some of these "grade grubbers" will argue for every little point on every exam. When it comes time for recommendations, you can bet professors will tell medical schools about the applicant's real personality.

On the other hand, letting professors or T.A.s get away with grading errors or unfairness is no good either. So, you should try to walk that fine line between being an over-aggressive jerk and being a piece of driftwood. By doing this, you can sometimes push your grade a little higher.

For example, don't be afraid during a lecture to ask the professor to explain a concept again. Better yet, ask the professor about it *after* class. It may turn up on the exam, and professors instinctively try to help students on material related to exam questions. When the student gets the question right, the professor feels he has done an excellent job teaching the material!

Also, get to know your teaching assistant. You don't have to be a brown-noser, but you should ask for help whenever you need it. If the T.A. sees that you're making a good effort, he'll be more willing to help you and may even boost your grade if you're on a borderline.

Finally, stand up for your rights. Tell your professor or T.A. if you think they are out of line (e.g. giving what you think is a bad test, not spending enough time on a difficult concept, etc.). Don't threaten them and don't whine, but talk to them in a rational and mature manner. You'll be surprised how interested they are in your opinion. They'll usually make changes or suggest methods to help you overcome your difficulty.

Pass/Fail Grades

An easy and enjoyable way to take a course is on a pass/fail basis. Unfortunately, competition for medical school makes taking your required premedical courses pass/fail unadvisable, because med schools have no way to interpret what a "pass" means in relation to your peers. Taking a few courses like sailing or drama pass/fail isn't a problem, but never take Organic pass/fail!

If you attend a college that uses a pass/fail system in lieu of all grades, request that your work be graded. It is unfortunate that stimulating learning experiences must be perverted into a scramble for grades, but that's the premedical reality.

Chapter 3

The MCAT

We cannot over-emphasize the importance of good MCAT scores. Though standardized tests continue to be criticized as culturally biased and dehumanizing, the MCATs remain the standard by which medical schools level grades from many different schools.

Nearly all medical schools require the MCAT. It's crucial that your scores be as high as possible, because at many med schools, *only* the combination of your grades and your MCAT scores determines whether you get an interview letter or a rejection letter. It's a very cold, "computer cut" process.

The moral of the story is simple: Don't treat lightly something that may mean as much as—if not more than—three years of grades combined.

MCAT Sections

The current MCAT, first given in 1991, consists of four sections, including a writing sample. The test lasts five hours, 45 minutes, but when you add a lunch break and the usual standardized testing delays, you'll be there about eight hours.

Section One of the exam, called **Verbal Reasoning** (a.k.a. "reading comprehension"), involves multiple-choice questions based on reading passages about 500 words long. The topics are selected at random from the humanities, social sciences, and natural sciences, and you're not expected to have any knowledge of the subjects.

People who do well on reading comprehension tests should have no trouble on this section. English majors, for example, will have a real advantage, since they have usually done more critical reading than the average science major. If you're anxious about this section, there's really only one solution: read more! But in the long run, you'll probably help yourself just as much by getting a good night's sleep and eating a light breakfast before the exam.

Section Two, **Physical Sciences**, consists of a mixture of physics and general chemistry questions. You're expected to answer the questions based on your knowledge of basic science concepts, plus your comprehension of the information presented in passages, graphs, and tables that accompany the questions. Unlike Section One, you can greatly improve your score in Section Two through intensive review of past course material.

After lunch, you get Section Three, the **Writing Sample**, which requires you to write two essays, each based on a quotation. You have 30 minutes for each essay, and in each you must first interpret the statement, then oppose the statement, and then resolve the conflict you've established. The key to this section is to remember that the graders are only expecting a first-draft effort. Don't get caught with an unfinished essay because you've been rewriting, revising, and polishing your interpretation. It's far more important to complete the three tasks in an organized, coherent fashion.

Section Three is made more challenging by the fact that it begins right after lunch. Often, people finish Section Two feeling very hungry, so they gorge themselves at lunch. Then they return to the testing room and start to feel drowsy, suffering from what we call *Food Coma*! By the time they've got to write the second essay, their minds have turned to mush.

The remedy for this is easy: don't eat large portions of red meat or greasy food at lunch. Instead, eat trail mix, salad, tuna, chicken, or other light fare.

If you don't stuff yourself during lunch and remain calm while writing, you shouldn't have overwhelming problems with Section Three.

Section Four, **Biological Sciences**, is identical in format to Section Two, except for two big differences. First, the questions are on biology and organic chemistry. Second, it's the last section of the test, and you'll undoubtedly be sick and tired of filling in those little bubbles with your #2 pencil.

The solution to the first problem is simple: study. The solution to the fatigue is a little sneakier. Bring something sugary, like a Snickers bar, in your pocket. (Technically, food is not allowed in the testing room, but who ever bothers with petty rules like that?) During Section Three, eat the candy. If you time it right, you should have a big sugar high to get you through the last section. So after the test you lapse into a Food Coma. But who cares? It's over!

It's important to remember that the MCAT is designed to break you and everyone else. The propaganda written by the test-makers will tell you that the MCAT will measure the "problem-solving" and "communication" skills necessary for your career as a physician. Maybe, but what it really measures is your endurance, which is probably the most important quality you need to be a doctor anyway.

With the MCAT you have no choice: you have to play their game, by their rules. But you can play it smart. Everyone knows it's just a weeder, so don't get hyper-anxious and let yourself become a weed that gets plucked.

Scoring the MCAT

The MCAT gives four scores, which reflect your performance in each section. The scores for Verbal Reasoning, Physical Sciences, and Biological Sciences are reported on a scale of 1 to 15 (with 15 as the highest). Your raw score—the actual number of correctly answered problems—is converted to this 1-15 scale so people who take different MCATs can be compared to one another.

Two readers grade each essay. The essays are scored "holistically," which can be best defined as "by gut feeling." You don't get one point for spelling, one point for sentence structure, one point for grammar, and so on. Instead, readers give a single score for their overall impression of the essay. However, your score will be automatically reduced if you don't address all three tasks required in each essay. The four essay scores (two per essay) are combined into one raw score, which gets converted to an alphabetical scale of J to T (with T as the highest).

Although your raw score may be lower than the raw score of someone who took the MCAT after you, your scaled score may be the same, because it reflects your performance among your peers—and that's the truly useful information. The test-makers assume that the 34,000 or so people who take the MCAT offer pretty much the same distribution of intelligence, anxiety, preparation, sleeplessness, etc. each time the test is given, and that no huge anomalies exist. Thus, the graders shift the bell curve to account for the variation in difficulty of individual MCATs but a uniformity in test-taking populations.

Many medical schools look for *consistency* in MCAT scores. If your three numerical scores are above 10, and your essay score is respectable, your chances of an interview are quite good. But two 14's on the science sections won't help if you got a 6 in Verbal Reasoning and your essay score reflects the fact that you drew pretty pictures on the paper.

Interestingly, studies have found little correlation between MCAT scores alone and good medical school performance. And high grades in med school don't guarantee you'll be a good physician, either. But medical schools will continue to use the MCAT to make decisions about applicants, so you're just going to have to deal with it.

Preparing for the MCAT

When you receive your MCAT registration packet from the Association of American Medical Colleges, you'll read on the second page of the instruction booklet something like, "The AAMC has conducted analyses comparing the performances of examinees who enroll in commercial review courses with those who do not (*yak, yak, yak, blah, blah, blah*), and we have found that gains derived from taking commercial review courses are small—only one-half of one scaled score point."

Now, this may sound like doing well on the MCAT has something to do with genetics or your intrinsic intelligence or something crazy like that. Well, that's simply bunk! The MCAT is not the SAT, and it's not about seeing three dimensional relationships in space like an I.Q. test. It's about getting concepts down in your head so they're as fresh as when you first learned them two or three years ago.

The point is, there are no curve balls on the MCAT, and studying for it, as for any other test, *will* boost your scores.

But there are no short cuts, either. Preparing for the MCAT requires a lot of diligence—and diligence is exactly what the MCAT measures! Getting high scores is really a function of how badly you want to get in, and in our opinion, how badly you want to get in is the most important piece of information an admissions committee can have about your potential success.

The earlier you start preparing, the better. Reviewing for the MCAT will involve effort as any other test—just much, much more. We recommend you start the review at least six (and probably nine) months before the exam. This doesn't mean reading an MCAT review book five minutes before you go to bed. You should start an intensive review of concepts and information that will be *pertinent* to the exam (see outline in *The MCAT Student Manual*).

We cannot stress enough the importance of focusing your study on relevant topics during this critical period. For example, don't start reviewing old notes from chemistry class, because you'll only get bogged down in an incredible amount of superfluous material. You'll end up studying information in a depth that you'll never see on the MCAT. (By the way, this skill of discriminating study will be essential in medical school, where you must decide what's important from a mind-boggling amount of information.)

Remember, the MCAT tests very basic concepts. Occasionally they are disguised in a somewhat complicated question, but usually they are given in a straightforward manner.

The problem is, there are many questions on a wide range of topics, so you may be asking yourself, "Well, how do I know what basic concepts to study and what to ignore?" Fortunately, someone has answered that question for you. Perhaps the most important investment you can make to get into medical school (besides this book, of course) is *A Complete Preparation for the MCAT* by James L. Flowers, M.D., M.P.H.(see the list of suggested readings at the end of the chapter). In his book, Dr. Flowers offers succinct review notes that parallel the outline of science topics in *The MCAT Student Manual*, which was written by the same people who devise the MCAT.

Get the idea? Dr. Flowers implies that if you know his book thoroughly, you should average a minimum of 11 in the science portions of the MCAT. From our personal experience, this is quite accurate.

Unfortunately, it's more difficult to increase your scores in the reading and writing sections, because they involve skills that you either have or have not developed in the course of your entire education. So don't sweat it! You can't worry about things you can't improve. Concentrate on what you most certainly can improve: your science scores.

Professional MCAT Prep Courses

What about professional preparatory courses like Stanley Kaplan, Bar/Bri, The Princeton Review, etc.? We recommend them, but you should realize that you'll get out of them only what you put into them.

Stanley Kaplan Testing Centers offer the most popular courses. Now, we all know Stan makes big bucks every year off a lot a premedical students, but for about $700 he'll do a lot more for your MCAT scores than $60,000 worth of private college will. Plus, his fee doesn't seem so large when you consider that you'll spend about $4,000 just *applying* to med school.

For most students, the in-class part of the Kaplan course is not worthwhile—they don't tell you anything you can't get on your own. What you're really buying are hundreds of simulated MCAT exams. Stan can go a little overboard with the depth of his exam questions, so if you're getting about 75% or 80% on his exams, you'll probably get 11's or 12's on the real MCAT.

We suggest you take all the Kaplan tests. Then, listen only to the recorded answers of the questions you got wrong. Finally, review the subject areas that gave you difficulty in the practice tests. This process alone will take three months to do thoroughly. We can't guarantee you'll see identical questions on the real MCAT you take, but you'll have solved so many similar problems that it'll be a real challenge for the test maker to write a question that doesn't resemble a problem you've already seen on a Kaplan test.

In any event, Kaplan's tests show you where you are weak, and they decrease your anxiety about the MCAT—probably their most valuable function.

Again, to get your money's worth from any prep course, take all the sample tests and review your preparatory booklets on a regular basis. Set aside a regular time each week for intensive preparation. If you do these things consistently about 20 hours a week, and begin six to nine months before the exam, almost nothing can stop you from getting good MCAT scores.

Examination Tips

Though some of the following suggestions may seem obvious, students often forget them under the pressures of an examination. Therefore, read through them before you take the MCAT to remind yourself of test-taking strategies, and remember to adhere to them even when the test is not going smoothly:

1. **Read all directions with great care.** It's ridiculous how many errors occur due to carelessness in reading directions and headings.

2. **Time is a limiting factor.** Remember this when you're tempted to leave a question unanswered, with the expectation of returning to it later. The best thing to do is mark your best guess for the moment and star the question so you can go back to it later if you have time.

3. **Be conscious of your allotted time.** You must budget your time for each of the sections on the exam, so take a watch to the test. According to the *The MCAT Student Manual*, your total score is a reflection of your right answers only. This means you aren't penalized for guessing, so always guess! Do not leave any bubbles blank. If you have 30 seconds left and 10 unanswered questions, just fill in the same letter (e.g. "b") for all of them.

4. **In the reading comprehension section, quickly read the questions** *before* **you read the passage.** This way, you'll recognize the sections in the passage that deal with the questions. Also, the

questions are usually in the same order as the information in the passage, except sometimes one question comes right away that you can't answer until you finish the passage. Knowing this, you can usually keep the next question in mind, read the passage until you come to the answer, and then move on. By doing this, you read the passage only once and save a lot of time.

5. **All questions in the reading comprehension section are based only on information in the passage.** Do not use your own knowledge to answer any questions. Base your answers solely on the information in the passage.

6. **Before starting each essay, write a very brief outline in the margin of the booklet.** If you start to get bogged down in the essay, refer to the outline and recall the key points you want to express. If you try to organize it all in your head, you probably won't write a clear essay.

7. **While working the science sections, rely on your fundamental understanding of chemistry, biology, and physics.** Most questions in the science sections deal exclusively with basic principles.

Suggested Reading

A Complete Preparation for the MCAT. James L. Flowers, M.D., M.P.H. Betz Publishing, Inc., P.O. Box 34631, Bethesda, MD 20827 (phone 301-340-0030 or toll free 800-634-4365). This is absolutely the best preparation for the science sections of the MCAT—and we don't even get a cut of the profits for saying so.

MCAT Student Manual. Mary H. Littlemeyer & Alan C. Mauney. Association of American Medical Colleges (Attn: Membership & Publication Orders, One Dupont Circle, N.W., Suite 200, Washington, D.C. 20036; phone 202-828-0400). Do not take the MCAT without this one! It contains an authentic sample MCAT, which will give you an excellent idea of what the test is like and the kind of scores you'll receive.

Medical School Admission Requirements. Association of American Medical Colleges (address above). The Bible!

Chapter 4

The Application Process

The closest to perfection a person ever comes is when he fills out a job application form. Stanley J. Randall

In the preceding chapters, we explained ways you can achieve your highest potential grade point average and MCAT score. After following these recommendations, the time will finally come for you to apply to medical schools, to show the various admissions committees why you should be allowed to enter their school. It is the most critical and, in some ways, the most difficult step.

You'll probably feel frustrated and cheated when you realize that you're expected to transfer years of preparation and effort onto four pieces of paper. While we agree this may not be the best way to evaluate an applicant, we are not writing a critique of the admissions process here. We just want to tell you how to work best within the system and how to make the system work for you. As far as admissions committees are concerned, you are *only* what your application says you are (until the interview), and you should use this fact to your advantage.

If admissions committees were able to live with applicants and see them as they really are, they'd probably reject most of them. So here's a flaw in the application process that works *for* you: those four sheets of paper are not very good at revealing what a person is really like. With a little effort, anyone can shine on an application.

Often, applicants are unsuccessful simply because they haven't mastered the ability to manipulate the process to their advantage as well as those who are successful. Our goal is to refine your skills of manipulation.

The two components of your application that are already set in stone are your grade point average and MCAT scores. You can't change them, so don't worry about them. Your "personal statement" (usually a biographical essay) and recommendations are items that you'll complete shortly before you send your application. (The end of this chapter has a concise timetable of events in the application process. Use it to mark your progress and keep track of important events.)

If you already have good grades, don't write anything in your essay that could give a bad impression (e.g., extremist political opinions, embarrassing intimate details, etc.). If your grades are not so great, the essay is your chance to show med schools what you're really made of. An excellent essay and glowing recommendations are the only items in the application over which you have control. Their careful execution is critical, and we will discuss them in greater detail shortly.

Remember, your application is the only "you" that medical schools will know. If they are impressed with the "you" on the application, they will want to see the real you for an interview.

AMCAS and the Application

Years ago, applying to medical school was an even more laborious task. Students had to fill out a separate application for every med school—a time-consuming process, as you can imagine.

Fortunately, the American Medical College Application Service (AMCAS) has simplified the application process. You can now send one application to AMCAS, which will forward copies to the schools you specify. Unfortunately, a few medical colleges are still not part of AMCAS, and you must request separate applications from each of these schools. As of this writing, the non-AMCAS schools are

Baylor University
Brown University
Columbia University
Harvard University
Johns Hopkins University
New York University

Texas A & M University
Texas Tech University
U. of Missouri, Kansas City
U. of North Dakota
U. of Rochester
U. of Tennessee, Memphis
U. of Texas (Dallas, Galveston, Houston, San Antonio)
Yale University

You'll find these schools' addresses in *Medical School Admission Requirements* (published by the Association of American Medical Colleges), which should be your Bible. It includes every essential piece of information on admission statistics and requirements you could possibly imagine. Get it. You will refer to it often.

AMCAS is just the first level of the application process. When you make it through AMCAS, you'll get a secondary application unique for each school. They range from a more detailed version of the AMCAS application to a simple request for more money "so we may further evaluate your application."

After the secondary application, you'll be asked for an interview. Rejection can come at any stage, but making it through AMCAS is the most important hurdle, because after AMCAS the process becomes a little more personal and subjective. It's easier to be "creative" post-AMCAS than in the pre-AMCAS, GPA-and-MCATs-only stage.

You can get an AMCAS application from your premedical advisor, from AMCAS medical schools, or from AMCAS directly at

AMCAS
Association of American Medical Colleges
Section for Student Services
2450 N St. N.W.
Washington, D.C. 20036-1989
(Phone: 202-828-0600)

Your application must include a check, which is AMCAS' fee for its distribution service. The amount depends on the number of schools to which you want your application sent. (For the 1993 entering class, the fee was $200 for six schools, and $10 for each school over six.) Then, the med schools will request about $50 extra when you receive their secondary application. You can waive some of these fees if you can demonstrate financial hardship.

You must also send an official transcript to AMCAS of all college work completed. You should request this from your school early, since many large schools are slow, and the delay will hold up the rest of your AMCAS application. Most medical schools ask you to put your last semester's grades on the back of their secondary application, saying they "won't get the latest transcripts in time." Actually, it's a sly way to test your integrity. Any discrepancy between the grades you report and official records will prompt the admissions committee to reject your applicaltion immediately.

You will not need to send your MCAT scores, since AMCAS is the same bunch that gave you the MCAT. How nice . . .

Both the AMCAS application and the secondary applications have deadlines. A golden rule in this game is to submit every application at the *earliest* allowed date. Many people think medical schools wait for all applications, make their selections, and reject the rest. Nothing could be further from the truth. Students are accepted on a **rolling basis**. In other words, every day after the earliest possible date you wait to send your application, you have less and less chance of being admitted. Many qualified applicants have been shocked into reality when they waited until the last minute to apply and found that no spaces remained.

Your Extracurricular Activities
A man may be so much of everything that he is nothing of anything. Samuel Johnson

Experience is not what happens to a man; it is what a man does with what happens to him. Aldous Huxley

Extracurricular activities are very important to your application—never believe otherwise—because they show medical schools things about you that your GPA and MCATs never will. Of course, med schools first want to know that you're intellectually competent, but they also want to see more than just scores and a high I.Q. Extracurricular activities demonstrate your personality, your motivation level, and even your basis for choosing medicine.

Before you say, "I want to be a doctor," it's crucial to know *why* you really mean it. Spending all your time making an A in Organic Chemistry will never tell you if medicine is your calling. Therefore, it's **imperative** that you go to a hospital and do some sort of medical work. If they won't employ you, then volunteer. You'll gain experience and knowledge, and you'll show medical schools that you're genuinely motivated and interested. When they ask, "So, Mr. Smith, why do you want to become a doctor?" you can say, "Well, for the past three years I've worked in an emergency room near campus, and I've found it rewarding and fascinating."

Similarly, if medical research is your thing, you can apply for summer work in a genetic engineering company or any firm engaged in biomedical research.

This way, you'll show that you've based your decision to enter medicine on practical, personal experience—experience that will impress admissions committees as to the validity and conviction of your statement. (*Note:* Most committees actually assign points to an applicant's file based on the breadth and depth of their medical-related work.)

The key concept is simple: get medical experience as an undergraduate, and make it your principal extracurricular activity. If you have an interest in a particular field of medicine, try to get work in that field. You might be surprised to learn that pediatrics, for example, isn't right for you after all. It's much better to find out early than ten years down the road, when it will be much harder to change professions.

If you don't have an interest in any specialty, don't be afraid to try anything in a hospital that will give you good experience. It may work out great, or it may bore you to tears. What's important is that it's a learning experience and a chance for you to check out the business, so to speak. Don't fool yourself by thinking that after you get accepted to medical school you'll have lots of time to decide what kind of doctor you want to be. You don't. So it's a good idea to start looking around in your college years, when making an incorrect choice won't hurt much.

If you can't find a position in a field that interests you, check in a service-related field. For example, drug counselor, resident advisor, suicide prevention hot-line volunteer, etc. are good options. These types of activities indicate your desire to help people, which is a very important point. Many applicants will talk about how much they want to "help humanity," yet their only extracurriculars are "fraternity social chairman" and "captain of co-ed water polo team." No wonder admissions committees treat them with skepticism.

Finally, extracurricular work totally unrelated to medicine may be fine also. If you do something that interests and intrigues your interviewers, you will stick out in their minds. After seeing 300 applicants, interviewers tend to view everyone as pretty similar.

For instance, if an applicant had average grades and MCAT scores and no relevant medical work—but she had won an Olympic medal—she'd probably land in medical school easily. Similarly, a college student who started his own pizza parlor or had a book published would also stand out from the pack. This doesn't mean you have to become an Olympic athlete or an entrepreneur. But if you want to do some kind of unique work, by all means do it. The main point: be interesting.

However, extracurricular activities should never come at the expense of your GPA. No amount of extracurriculars will be an excuse for poor grades. Also, it's not necessary for you to list thousands of extracurriculars on your application. A few impressive activities in which you are genuinely involved count more than a deluge of "So what?" activities.

By now, most of you probably are wondering what you can do *this year* to put on your application. Well, you literally can do hundreds of things. All schools have clubs. (But don't think that just because there's a premedical club you should join it. Medical schools are rarely impressed with them.) Join a club that applies to your major. Becoming a club officer always looks impressive because it shows leadership potential—an important quality for many physicians. Being an athlete is also great. Anyone who can maintain a schedule of rigorous practice and studying and still keep good grades deserves to be commended. A student government office is good for similar reasons. Community volunteer work always looks good. Help out at a soup kitchen or with a literacy program, or join Big Brothers/Big Sisters.

If your school does any research at all, you should be able, with a little effort, to start working with a professor in his lab. If you are really lucky and dedicated, you may even get your name on a publication. This is extremely impressive! You might even consider being a teaching assistant in a course.

As for summer work, many universities and their medical schools sponsor programs designed especially for the undergraduate who wants hands-on experience. It's no secret that many people are admitted to medical schools through "back doors" like these. The programs offer a great opportunity for you to work for, and get to know, someone on the med school's admissions committee. It doesn't guarantee you'll get in, of course, but a personal contact can't hurt. Medical schools will send you the relevant information on these programs, which often provide a stipend for living expenses.

Finally, if all you can do in the summer is work in a regular job (waitress, delivery man, working for your dad, etc.) because you need the money, then that's what you need to do. Just be sure to make your reasons clear in your application.

Recommendations

I don't care what is written about me, so long as it isn't true.
Katharine Hepburn

Recommendations are one of the most important factors in the selection of medical students. Therefore, like the MCAT, you must not take them lightly.

Many applicants don't start thinking about recommendations until junior year, when they're due. Ideally, though, you should start to think about them from Day One of *freshman* year! Students also mistakenly assume that the person who writes your recommendation is going to write a good one. Instead, you must constantly think, "Do my professors really know me, or am I just another body in the classroom?" When the time comes to ask your professors for recommendations and they don't even know your name, you'll be in deep trouble.

We all know the students constantly blathering in class—and

everyone wishes they would just shut up. Well, those are people the professor remembers, too, so try to be like them—but don't be pushy and obnoxious to the point that you're remembered in a negative way. Simply be inquisitive and sound interested. Try to see your professors in their office hours and ask only a few questions to clarify major points in class. You may be surprised to find that the subject matter becomes more interesting when you force yourself to look at the material hard enough to ask intelligent questions. If your questions are intricate, save them until after the lecture. Your professor will be impressed by the depth of your understanding and appreciate your not interrupting the flow of the lecture.

Ask only "clarification" questions in class. Don't publicly correct the professor when he is wrong, but don't hesitate to do so later in the form of a question. He'll announce the correction in the next class and remember your brilliance in his recommendation letter.

A good recommendation should reflect more than just a casual acquaintance. It should also carry some weight—the more the better. You don't need to solicit Nobel laureates, but a little strategic thinking beforehand about whom you will ask can do wonders to enhance your appeal to medical schools.

A professor should be able to say more about you than, "She received a grade of A in my class." Therefore, when you ask a professor for a recommendation, ask first if he thinks he can write you a good one. Tell him to be totally honest. It's the only way to get an idea of what he'll write, since you should always request to have a closed file. (A "closed file" means you are not allowed to look at what was written about you. It's the only way to get honest, credible letters, since a professor is likely to be less candid if he knows you can read what he wrote later. This goes for both praise and criticism.)

Further, to give the admissions committee a more balanced profile, choose professors from different fields (i.e., don't get recommendations from only your chemistry professor buddies).

A recommendation from the professor with whom you do research is great because it might tell an admissions committee about your lab expertise *and* how well you work with others.

A letter from the physician who oversees your volunteer work is also valuable, because it might describe how you deal with sick people. Sometimes, it's even a good idea to have a teaching assistant who knows you well write the recommendation, and then have the professor co-sign it (only the prof's signature gives the letter any weight).

Letters of recommendation from family, friends, graduate students, medical students, and high school teachers are not acceptable. They only indicate poor judgment by the applicant.

In the past, it was common practice to ask a professor directly for a recommendation to send to medical schools. Today, that practice has been supplanted by a **composite recommendation**, where a premedical committee at your college drafts a letter of recommendation from letters written by people of your choice. This means that getting to know your premedical advisor is a very good idea. This also means that if the premedical committee can't write a good letter, it doesn't matter how good the rest of your letters were.

You can't do much about the composite letter, so don't worry about it. If the committee can't write well, your only consolation is that everybody else in your school is in the same boat. However, most composite letters include direct quotes from the professor's letters. The composite letter also ranks you in comparison to your peers in motivation, integrity, sincerity, and leadership. In addition, the letter usually begins by saying how "competitive this undergraduate institution is, and how hard it is to get good grades at this great school, etc. . . ."

Because it's all so subjective, most admissions committees ignore the bull and go straight to the quotes. Therefore, you should strongly suggest that your premedical committee include such quotes—and even the actual letters from your recommenders.

In short, the composite method has some pitfalls, but try to use it to your advantage, and never make an enemy of anyone. You never know who will serve on the premedical committee.

Filling Out the Application

An autobiography usually reveals nothing bad about the writer except his memory. Franklin P. Jones

Since the application is your chance to tell medical schools why you are so special, give it a lot of extra care.

The first rule: type it neatly. Never use a dot matrix printer. In fact, many students actually pay money to have their essay professionally typeset, but that's probably going overboard. A high quality laser printer will make it look great, however.

Rule #2: the application should be totally perfect. A simple typographical error may be reason enough to reject someone when there are thousands of applicants to weed out.

Finally, don't even *consider* having someone else write your essay, let alone paying for such a service. Such "professional" essays are always too good to be true and will certainly raise some eyebrows. They may get you some interviews, but if your verbal skills resemble a punch-drunk boxer rather than William F. Buckley, you'll be out! Anyway, after four years of sweat, is that *really* the way you want to get into medical school?

Don't forget all the jobs you've held in the past few years. Many applicants never include some jobs because they think only work related to health-care is significant. But any job shows a willingness to work—a trait you'll need in abundance in medical school. Besides, leaving out miscellaneous work experiences may result in that section of the application looking very empty.

Further, you never know what the person who reads your application is looking for, so include all your jobs. A member of an admissions committee told us a story that illustrates this point: An applicant's essay made the student sound so arrogant that the admissions officer was just about to toss the whole thing. Then, he noticed that the student had worked a summer in construction. He wondered how someone so arrogant could do that kind of job. Intrigued, he decided to interview him. It turned out the student wasn't at all the way he sounded in his essay, and he was admitted.

You should also include all the honors you've achieved. Most people have something to put in this section, and it becomes not a question of "What's there?" but rather, "Is *something* there?"

Many people initially think they have no honors, but when they think harder they realize they have a few awards to write in. Remember, never leave a section blank.

The key thing is, you're supposed to tell your life story on the application. In other words, you're describing how you spend your time. If you spend time climbing mountains, playing the flute, ballooning, singing opera, skydiving, surfing, or anything that's just plain out of the ordinary, let them know. Medical schools always like to say how interesting and diverse their students are. They just love it if you do something eccentric or unique—and you probably do if you think about it for a while.

How Many Schools Should You Apply To?

There are three kinds of lies: lies, damned lies, and statistics.
Benjamin Disraeli

Applying to medical school can be very expensive. You must pay for the AMCAS application, the secondary applications, and then transportation and accommodations when you interview. But compared to the cost of a medical education, the application expense is trivial, and you should never let money limit the number of schools to which you apply.

If you can demonstrate financial hardship, the AMCAS (and sometimes the secondary application) fees can be waived. However, most students do not fall in the extremely low family income level that's required for a waiver, even though you may be receiving financial aid at college. Often, medical schools will help reduce your expenses by letting you stay with a medical student when you interview.

But even after cutting lots of corners, you're still looking at a cost somewhere between $1,000-$5,000, depending on how many schools you apply to. That may sound outrageous, but consider what your undergraduate education will cost—probably $30,000-$100,000—then add the potential cost of med school—another $60,000 to $100,000. Compared to this, even a large application budget is fairly insignificant.

Therefore, it doesn't matter whether you must beg or borrow—you should *never* let financial matters become a limiting factor in your application to medical school. Years of expensive work and planning should not go down the drain for such a minor reason.

So the question becomes, "How many schools should I apply to?" There's no easy answer, but consider the following: The average medical school receives about 5,000 applications for 100 positions. If the selection process were entirely random, your chance of being accepted would be one-in-50 (2%). To put it in a more depressing way, your chance of being rejected would be 98%. Sounds pretty dismal, doesn't it?

But wait. If you apply to a number of schools, your chance of being accepted by at least one school is one minus your chance of being rejected by all of the schools. That is,

$$\% \text{ ACCEPTANCE} = 1-(.98)N \times 100$$

where N is the number of schools to which you apply. Let's plug in some sample numbers:

N =	% Acceptance =
1	2
5	10
10	18
20	33
30	45

In reality, of course, the process is not totally random, though there are random elements in it. The point is, even if you're a straight-A student, it would be unwise to apply to fewer than five schools. Basically, the more the better. If you are a really strong student, you should apply to no fewer than ten. If you're like most people, 20 and even 30 schools would be a good idea.

Many applicants don't realize that applying to as many schools as possible is as important as doing well in school or on the MCAT. Of course, you must never compromise quality for quantity of applications.

The 2% probability of acceptance at a particular medical school is not really as bad as it sounds. First, approximately 34,000 students apply each year for approximately 17,000 positions. So, your actual overall probability of being accepted to at least one medical school (if you apply across the board) is about 50%.

Not bad. The figure of 2% comes from the fact that every applicant applies to more than one school, giving the illusion that there are more applicants than available positions. Therefore, your chance of being accepted to at least one medical school after applying to 20 is actually higher than 33%, because the number of applicants is much less than the number of applications received by medical schools.

Our goal here is not to turn you into a statistician or a gambler, but to stress the point that all the hard work in the world won't get you in if you don't apply intelligently. You must be fully aware of how to increase your odds—which usually means submitting as many applications as possible.

Deciding Where To Apply

Students with high grades and MCAT scores will likely have a wide choice of medical schools to attend. However, they are a minority, because most students usually get accepted to only one or two schools. Therefore, it's critical that you choose the correct schools to which to apply.

We recommend that you divide the number of schools you plan to apply to into quarters and rank them on their relative appeal. (The end of the chapter has a ranking of schools.) The first quarter should include schools where you never expect to get accepted but would attend instantly if you did (e.g. Harvard). The second quarter should include the very competitive schools, then the strong schools, and the final fourth should be last-choice schools.

For example, if you apply to 20 schools, you would choose five schools from each of the four groups at the end of the chapter. By spreading yourself out like this, you'll increase your odds of acceptance and maybe get some nice surprises.

You should consider whether the school is public or private. In general, public schools accept mostly state residents, so applying to the Univ. of Tennessee when you live in Connecticut could be a total waste of time.

On the other hand, such a rule can work to your advantage. In some states, especially in the midwest, the number of in-state applicants is so small that the public medical schools have trouble filling their classes. Therefore, nearly every state resident who applies gets in, so the admission requirements are much lower than at private schools. If you move to one of these states and establish residency, you have an almost sure acceptance to the state medical school. Of course, this ploy is drastic and should be a last resort.

Another thing to determine is the school's acceptance ratio (how many students it accepts versus how many apply). Of course, you'll want to look for the largest ratio. *Medical School Admission Requirements* will have all this data.

Other important questions to consider:

1. **Do you like the location?** Although you'll probably attend whatever med school you get in—and you should never eliminate schools in your state of residence—it doesn't hurt to at least consider location before applying. There are many medical schools in many different locales, so you shouldn't have to settle for a place where you'll be miserable.

2. **What are the school's facilities like?** This is very important, because it will give you an indication of what types of patients you'll see and how many you'll see. In general, county and city hospitals see much more action than private hospitals. The number of patients the hospital treats annually will also indicate how much clinical experience you'll get. If you want to become involved in research, find out the amount and type of research conducted at that school.

3. **How is the education delivered?** Find out how many days per week—and how many hours per day—you're in school. Most medical schools go five days a week; some go four or six. Some have nine hours of class per day; others average only four. Some schools provide note-taking services; others make you struggle on your own. Some ease the tension by having a pass/fail grading system; others can be cutthroat and neurotic with letter grades. The curriculum may not seem important to you now, when all you're thinking about is "Will I get in?", but these points are critical, because they can make the difference between an exciting learning experience and a miserable one.

Financial Aid for Medical School

It sounds implausible, but it's totally true: your finances should not restrict your choice of medical school. Once you are accepted, the school will work with you to insure that you and your family will be able to pay tuition and still live well.

All medical schools inform students about the Guaranteed Student Loan (GSL), Health Education Assistance Loan (HEAL), Supplemental Loan for Students (SLS), Perkins Loan, Homan Loan, University Loans, and other state programs. Note also the federally-funded Armed Forces Scholarship and the Medical Scientist Training Program (MSTP)—it's open to all students and pays tuition plus stipend (see below for more information). First- and second-year minority students get information about the National Medical Fellowships.

There are lots more scholarship and loan programs—too many to list here. The bottom line is, your medical school's financial aid office will help you meet the high cost of your education.

Don't worry about signing for loans, either. You'll be able to repay the loans for your tuition pretty easily—and eventually you might have enough left over to buy Mom and Dad a nice Mercedes-Benz. Skeptical? To convince you, we've listed below the 1991 nonacademic median salaries of the various specialties as reported in the *Physician Compensation Survey Report* by the Center for Research in Ambulatory Health Care Administration and the Medical Group Practice Association:

Specialty	Median compensation
Anesthesiologist	$220,800
Cardiologists (invasive)	$258,875
Cardiovascular surgeon	$420,090
Dermatologist	$145,092
Emergency medicine	$123,942
Family practicioner	$101,876
Gastroenterologist	$188,133
General surgeon	$172,952
Internist	$110,606
Neurologist	$132,000
Neurosurgeon	$338,692

Ob/Gyn	$197,745
Orthopedic surgeon	$274,255
Pediatrician	$104,937
Psychiatrist	$110,143
Pulmonologist	$154,795
Radiologist	$246,462
Urologist	$195,715

Since we have raised the issue of earning potential, we feel we should remind you that good medicine always requires the doctor to place the patient's needs first. If your goal is to make a ton of money in as little time as possible, go into investment banking. You'll be happier and society will benefit more. If your concern is how you're ever going to repay medical school loans, relax. You may have to wait a little longer than your business school friends to buy a house or go to Hawaii, but if you're enjoying your profession, it's well worth it.

Final Review of Your Application
A few more points to consider before you mail that AMCAS application:

1. Make a final check for absolute, 100% neatness.

2. Have other people read what you've written. Your premedical advisor, a premedical friend, or the family physician are good choices, since they are familiar with the process. An English teacher can help with style or grammar problems.

3. Make sure you use the entire space (with reasonably sized print and margins, of course) for personal comments, and try to be original. For example, don't write about how you've wanted to be a doctor since you were a kid. This was everyone's ambition at age four. Most applicants will spend months working on their essay before they write the final version, so get started way in advance. We'll discuss the essay in greater depth in Chapter 6.

4. Photocopy the application and keep it in a safe place in case AMCAS loses it, and also for interview preparation.

5. Always send the application via certified mail if you are ap-

proaching a deadline. This will put the burden of explanation on AMCAS should the application be lost.

After You've Applied

Once you file your application, it will be just a matter of time before you receive requests for interviews. In the meantime, it's important that you follow up on your application.

For starters, keep a meticulous record of your status at each school. We recommend making a chart with your schools in one column, receipt of application, secondary application, interview, etc. in other columns. Write in the date when each category is filled. This way, you'll know if a school seems overdue for a note or phone call from you.

As for phoning schools, it's perfectly acceptable. Of course, you don't what to harass them, but calling occasionally to determine the status of your application is a good idea, since applications do get lost and letters of recommendation misplaced. If you try to be extremely cordial on the phone, you may find yourself on a first-name basis with the secretaries. This may sound unimportant, but one applicant got to know the secretary well enough that she hand-carried his application to the Dean of Admissions at U.C. Davis.

If you're not accepted right away, don't panic and ruin your senior year of college. Some applicants will receive acceptance letters in the fall, but don't expect to be accepted until the spring.

Often, half of an entering medical class comes from the waiting list, so don't get discouraged if you are wait-listed. If several schools do put you on a waiting list, the odds are good you'll get into at least one, since these lists are usually about twice as large as the actual entering class.

As you wait to hear from schools, have an answering machine or someone always available to receive messages, especially as you approach the end of summer and the beginning of medical school registration.

Also, keep the admissions department abreast of any extra awards, publications, etc. which may strengthen your application. (However, sending new transcripts, unless they are dramatically improved, is usually not helpful.) Here's a good example:

A student had planned to matriculate at his second-choice school. The week before classes began, he was in the newspaper for placing third in a balloon race in Allentown, PA. He mailed the article to his first-choice school and drew an arrow to himself in the newspaper photograph saying, "Please, pick me up!" The school called him the day before classes began and offered him admission. After partying on Bourbon Street in New Orleans, he sped north to New York City—another happy ending . . .

Handling Acceptances

Students usually begin collecting letters of acceptance at their safety schools first. According to the rules of the game, applicants may not hold more than two acceptance offers unless they are waiting to compare financial aid packages.

This rule can make things tricky. For example, one applicant was holding acceptance to four schools when a Director of Admissions threatened to retract his acceptance if the applicant didn't decide soon. (All AMCAS-participating schools know your status at the other schools to which you applied.) After being confronted, the student rushed to the post office and declined admission at three of the four schools. For the fourth school, he quickly filled out and mailed the registration form weeks early—thereby committing himself to that school.

A few days later, Johns Hopkins (a better school than any of the original four that had accepted him) learned that the applicant was now holding only one spot, and they offered him a place. Unfortunately, Johns Hopkins had to retract the offer when they discovered that the student had officially registered at another school.

The lesson: don't hold multiple acceptances, but don't rush to register at any school early.

Special Programs*

Medical Scientist Training Program (MSTP): The National Institutes of Health (NIH) provides funding to students who wish to pursue scientific and medical training (M.D.-Ph.D.) at the 25 schools listed below. Each year, approximately 140 students receive scholarships that pay a stipend and full tuition. After training, the student is obligated to conduct research or teach, usually for five years.

(Another 80 schools provide the option of obtaining the M.D.-Ph.D degree also, but these are not funded by the NIH. Some of these programs are funded privately; others are not funded at all. Information on these programs usually comes with the school's application.)

The NIH-supported programs are at these schools:

Albert Einstein	U.C. San Diego
Baylor	U.C. San Francisco
Case Western Reserve	U. of Iowa
Chicago-Pritzker	U. of Michigan
Columbia	U. of Minnesota
Cornell	U. of Pennsylvania
Duke	U. of Pittsburgh
Emory	U. of Rochester
Harvard	U. of Texas, Dallas
Johns Hopkins	U. of Virginia
Mount Sinai	U. of Washington
New York U.	Vanderbilt
Northwestern	Washington U. (St. Louis)
Stanford	Yale
UCLA	

B.A./B.S.-M.D. Programs: A few medical schools offer select high school students the opportunity to combine their undergraduate and medical training. The program, usually six years, lets students avoid much of the anxiety of the medical school application process.

*Data from Medical School Admissions Requirements, 1992-93, *published by the Association of American Medical Colleges.*

Albany Medical College
Boston U.
Brown
Case Western Reserve
City U. of New York*
Chicago—Pritzker
Eastern Tennessee State
Hahnemann (Philadelphia)
Howard (Washington DC)
Louisiana State*
Medical College of Pennsylvania
Medical College of Wisconsin
New York U.
Northeastern Ohio
Northwestern

Robert Wood Johnson
 (UMDNJ)
SUNY Brooklyn
SUNY Stonybrook
Thomas Jefferson
 (Philadelphia)
U.C. Irvine
UCLA
U. of Miami
U. of Michigan
U. of Missouri, Kansas
 City
U. of South Alabama
U. of Wisconsin, Madison*
Washington U. (St. Louis)

Program limited to state residents.

M.D.-J.D. Programs: This combined program allows medical students to pursue a law degree as well as their M.D. The following schools offer this program:

Duke
Southern Illinois U.
U. of Chicago

U. of Illinois
U. of Pennsylvania
Yale

Timetable of Important Dates

Junior Year

November through April: Begin review for MCATs.

February or March: Apply for spring MCAT.

April: Think about which medical schools to apply to. Collect letters of recommendation. Pick up AMCAS application packet. Suggested time to take MCAT.

May: Interpret MCAT scores and GPA with premedical advisor (see note below). Make first draft of AMCAS essay. Send for medical school catalogues. Send transcripts to AMCAS and non-AMCAS schools. Request the AMCAS application packet from

> American Medical College Application Service
> Association of American Medical Colleges
> Section for Student Services
> 2450 N Street N.W.
> Washington, DC 20036-1989
> (Phone: 202-828-0600)

June: Revise and polish AMCAS essay. Submit AMCAS application at earliest allowed date. Begin completing non-AMCAS applications as soon as possible.

August: Inform premedical committee where to send your composite recommendation letter (if your school has such a committee). Register for fall MCAT if scores were low and you feel you are better prepared.

Senior Year

September: Make sure all applications are complete and letters of recommendation received. Call to confirm if necessary. Fall MCAT offered.

November: Be patient. Interviews will come!

December: Try to schedule interviews during Winter Break for convenience.

January: Fill out GAPSFAS form for financial aid. Send updated transcripts if requested by schools.

February: If no one loves you by Valentines Day, speak immediately with your premedical advisor. He or she may be able to call on your behalf.

March: If you are wait-listed, send a letter expressing continued interest.

April and August: Acceptance letters are still sent out, so stay calm. Make sure medical schools can reach you or a family member by telephone at all times.

Note: Keep in mind that a few undergraduate pre-med programs like to boast "our acceptance rate to medical school is 80%" because it sounds impressive to high school students. (That is, students are more willing to pay the high tuition the school demands because they think they'll definitely get into medical school from that school.)

In reality, the acceptance rate is so high because the school does a premedical student weed-out. They tell mediocre students that their chances of getting into medical school are horrible, so they shouldn't even apply (when in fact they may have a reasonable chance of acceptance). So the only students who apply are stars who will get in easily—thus giving the high acceptance rate.

The lesson here is simple: take your premedical advisor's counseling with a grain of salt. The ultimate decisions should be yours alone.

Breakdown of U.S. Medical Schools*

The medical schools below are divided into quarters to help you make a rational decision about which schools to apply to. (Schools in Groups II and III are alphabetized within the group, not ranked.) See text for advice on choosing schools based on this grouping.

Group I: The Top Ten

(in order, according to *U.S. News & World Report*, March 23, 1992.)

1. Harvard University
2. Johns Hopkins University
3. Duke University
4. University of California—San Francisco †
   Yale University †
5. University of Pennsylvania
6. Washington University (St. Louis)
7. Stanford University
8. Columbia University
9. Cornell University
10. University of Michigan

† indicates a tie

Group II: Very Competitive

Baylor College of Medicine
Boston University School of Medicine
Indiana University School of Medicine
New York University School of Medicine
Northwestern University School of Medicine
Ohio State University College of Medicine
State University of New York at Buffalo School of Medicine
Temple University School of Medicine
Tufts University School of Medicine
Tulane University School of Medicine
University of California, Davis
University of California, Los Angeles

Information based on The Gourman Report, *National Education Standard, Los Angeles, CA, 1989.*

University of California, San Diego
University of Chicago, Pritzker School of Medicine
University of Illinois College of Medicine
University of Iowa College of Medicine
University of Minnesota Medical School
University of North Carolina School of Medicine
University of Rochester School of Medicine & Dentistry
University of Virginia School of Medicine
University of Washington School of Medicine
University of Wisconsin Medical School
Vanderbilt University School of Medicine

Group III: Competitive
Albany Medical College
Albert Einstein College of Medicine of Yeshiva University
Bowman Gray School of Medicine
Brown University Program in Medical Sciences
Case Western Reserve University School of Medicine
Creighton University School of Medicine
Dartmouth Medical School
Emory University School of Medicine
Georgetown University School of Medicine
George Washington University School of Medicine
Loma Linda University School of Medicine
Louisiana State University School of Medicine
Loyola University of Chicago Stritch School of Medicine
Michigan State University College of Human Medicine
Mount Sinai School of Medicine
Saint Louis University School of Medicine
State University of New York at Stony Brook
University of California, Irvine
University of Colorado School of Medicine
University of Connecticut School of Medicine
University of Florida College of Medicine
University of Kansas School of Medicine
University of Louisville School of Medicine
University of Maryland School of Medicine
University of Miami School of Medicine

University of Missouri School of Medicine, Columbia
University of Missouri School of Medicine, Kansas City
University of Oregon Medical School
University of Pittsburgh School of Medicine
University of Southern California
University of Texas, Dallas
University of Texas, Galveston
University of Texas, San Antonio
University of Utah College of Medicine
Wayne State University School of Medicine

Group IV: Good Schools
Everything else.

The Nation's Best Hospitals *

Johns Hopkins Hospital, *Baltimore, MD*

Mayo Clinic, *Rochester, MN*

Massachusetts General, *Boston, MA*

UCLA Medical Center, *Los Angeles, CA*

Cleveland Clinic, *Cleveland, OH*

Brigham & Women's Hospital, *Boston, MA*

Memorial Sloan-Kettering Cancer Center, *New York, NY*

Duke University Hospital, *Durham, NC*

Stanford University Hospital, *Stanford, CA*

UCSF, *San Francisco, CA*

* *According to* U.S. News & World Report, *August 5, 1991.*

Chapter 5

The Interview

If you think before you speak, the other fellow gets in his joke first. Ed Howe

The real art of conversation is not only to say the right thing in the right place, but to leave unsaid the wrong thing at the tempting moment. Dorothy Nevill

A good conversationalist is not one who remembers what was said, but says what someone wants to remember.
John Mason Brown

For applicants with good grades and MCAT scores, the interview is often just a formality. But for most students, it is a critical part of the admissions process.

The purpose of the interview is to obtain information independent of and supplementary to the data you supplied on the application. An interviewer may assess a candidate's academic potential, maturity, motivation, leadership, interests, knowledge of medicine, attitude, ability to relate to others, and other subjective criteria. A strong interview can increase your chance of admission tremendously, and a bad one can destroy even the class valedictorian. Therefore, it's essential that you understand what makes a good interview.

We believe interviewing is a skill you can learn. But, of course, it's impossible for us to teach you to interview well through a book. Improvement requires personal interaction. For example, if you think you may come across as shy, arrogant, or whatever, ask a friend or your premedical advisor to conduct mock interviews with you. It's an excellent way to improve your interviewing skills.

Better yet, use a video camera and VCR to study yourself as you answer questions. The tape will give you a realistic picture of how others perceive you. There are even courses designed to teach interviewing skills, but don't bother taking them unless you have a major problem (i.e. extreme shyness) to overcome.

The Interview Process

In general, the interview process is divided into three parts: the orientation, the tour, and the actual interview.

Not every school offers an orientation, but most do. Its purpose is not to evaluate applicants, but to inform them about what the day will entail.

All the other applicants to be interviewed will be with you at the orientation. Some may try to give you the impression that they are totally superior or that they were Albert Einstein in a past life or something. Don't pay any attention to them. They're just playing mind games with you and trying to mess with their competition. Just remain pleasant and smile a lot. Your display of maturity will probably bug them more than anything else you could do.

Use the orientation as a time to relax and gather your thoughts. Remember, if you are asked for an interview, it means they want you as much as you want them. Their goal for that day will be to sell you on their school and convince you to attend it over other schools that might accept you.

The Tour

After the orientation, you'll take a tour of the medical school. The tour, which will cover the clinical and instructional facilities, is when you'll get the big sales pitch. Many applicants get so anxious about their interview that they forget that the medical school is really the one under scrutiny. Contrary to popular opinion, one medical school is not like the next. Each school has a unique personality, which you may or may not like.

A medical student who has no bearing whatsoever on admissions decisions usually gives the tour, so feel free to ask any questions. It's essential that you take time in the tour to get a feel for the school, in case you must decide between two or more schools.

For this reason, unless lack of funds totally prohibits travel, never accept the option to be interviewed in your area rather than at the school. Many schools send a representative to, say, California to interview applicants who can't afford (or just don't want) to fly east.

If you can, spend the night before the interview with a medical student. He/she will usually offer good insight about what things are really like at the school.

The Interview

Your interviewers will be either two faculty members or one faculty member and one medical student. In the latter case, the faculty member will carry more weight, but don't underestimate the input from the student. Acting like he/she is a peon in the admissions process will guarantee your rejection. The faculty interview may help you get in, while the medical student interview can weed you out.

Again, either or both may be on the admissions committee, so it's not a good idea to say anything way out in left field. Instead, the interview is your chance to expand on information that may not be clear to the admissions committee. Applications do not have enough room for detail, and they force the applicant to abbreviate and oversimplify. Just remember to be yourself, since it's usually easy for an experienced interviewer to tell if someone is lying or exaggerating.

Many people tell horror stories of how a "friend of a friend" had some doctor give a him a really hard time in an interview. Of course, it's possible you'll encounter a jerk, but the fact is, most interviewers want to make the experience as stress-free as possible. Don't forget—the interviewer has been through the same thing and will be aware of (and usually sympathetic to) your nervousness.

One of our classmates did have a real hard time in one interview. At the end, the doctor said, "Sorry I was so hard on you, but it's only because I really want to recommend you. I wanted to be sure you had the right stuff. If I don't want somebody, I usually just give him a real easy interview."

So don't try to judge what somebody thinks of you by the way they treat you in the interview. Sometimes, they just want to see how you react to a stressful situation.

For example, there's an interviewer at one of the Texas schools who shakes your hand, smiles pleasantly, and asks, "So, how many times a week do you masturbate?" A friend of ours answered, without missing a beat, "Not as much as I deserve." Another friend was asked, "So, when are you going to get married?" To which she replied, "Is this a proposal?" Yet another female friend was asked, "Once you get married, how will your husband feel about your palpitating another man's scrotum?" Her reply was calm and professional.

Interviewers ask such questions only to see how you react to very personal or taboo subjects. Reacting with humor or a gentle response is far wiser than getting angry or upset. Remember, a physician must handle complex moral and ethical issues—and all types of patients—in a mature, tactful manner.

Then there are interviewers who just like to hear themselves talk. They want to impress you with how much they think they know. All you have to do is be a good listener, seem interested, and be patient. It'll be over soon.

Finally, if you don't know an answer to a question, just say, "I don't know." Nothing sounds worse than someone fumbling to make up an answer.

Final Preparation Before the Interview

You probably know the cliché, "You only get one chance to make a first impression." And given the volume of applicants that interviewers must see, the first impression is often the *only* impression. This means that for men, a suit, and for women, a conservative dress, are mandatory. And don't neglect personal grooming. Get a haircut, trim your beard, clean your fingernails, etc. We don't mean to sound like your Mom, but the informality of dorm life at college can make you forget how people dress and behave in the real world.

Before the interview, review your photocopy of the application you sent to the school. Often, interviewers will ask you to clarify or elaborate on something in your application. Chances are, you filled it out two months ago, and if you don't review it beforehand, you probably won't remember what the point was. This looks bad.

Also, read the catalog the school has sent you. Having a little substantive knowledge about the school looks impressive.

Above all, remember to pronounce the interviewer's name correctly, since you'll want to say, "Thank you, Dr. Radiziewski. It's been a pleasure speaking with you," or whatever. No sound is more important to people than the sound of their own names. In medical school interviews and in life in general, always refer to people by their names. It makes them feel, consciously or subconsciously, important—and they'll remember your kindness.

Being polite and personal also helps with the secretaries in the admissions office. More than one applicant has been derailed by being rude to the secretary. The secretary often attends the final admissions committee meeting, and since she has met *all* the applicants, she may occasionally make a negative statement—guaranteed to sink that applicant. No medical college wants a student who brown-noses professors and physicians while treating nurses, secretaries, and administrators with contempt. Besides, being on a first-name basis with the secretaries can help tremendously when you are curious about the status of your application.

Sample Interview Questions

Your interviewers will ask a variety of questions, and your answers should demonstrate your maturity, character, knowledge, and ability to communicate. There's really no way to "study" for an interview, but for curiosity's sake, we've compiled a list of questions asked in actual interviews. You may not get similar questions, but it might be useful just for practice to think about how you would answer them.

How do you know that medicine is for you?

What has been your most important accomplishment?

Do you think doctors are viewed with as much awe as in the past?

Is medicine becoming more technical, and is this beneficial?

What do you think of euthanasia? Abortion?

What do you think about the current proposals for a national health-care system?

What can be done about rising health-care costs?

What are your strong points? What are your weaknesses?

Do you have any hobbies?

Tell us about yourself.

Are you interested in any specialties?

What will you do if you don't get accepted to medical school?

Why do you want to work with sick people?

Do you think doctors are overpaid?

Do you feel you are prepared to enter medical school?

Why did you apply to this school? What other schools did you apply to? Why?

How will you finance your education?

Tell us about your undergraduate institution.

When did you decide to become a doctor?

Would you consider applying to a foreign medical school if you were rejected by all the U.S. schools?

Are quotas fair?

Are you concerned about the surplus of doctors that's supposed to occur when you begin practicing?

What makes you different from everyone else?

What do you know about AIDS? How do you feel about treating HIV-positive patients?

What three adjectives best describe you?

What do you see yourself doing 10 years from now? (*A very popular question. Unfortunately, one student answered, "Uh, this is Wednesday, about two o'clock, right?" The interviewer said, "Yes, it is." As he swung his arm up as if he were holding a golf club, he said, "I should be on the eighth hole." Apparently, his humor wasn't appreciated—he was rejected by that school.*)

Where would you want to go to medical school, given the choice?

How do you intend to integrate medical school (or your medical practice) and your family/social life?

What do you do for fun?

Describe your relationship with your mother/father/siblings.

What do you know about hospices, HMOs, or PPOs?

How do you think malpractice will affect you?

What do you expect to get from medicine?

Do you have any children, or plan to? (*This is actually an illegal question, because female applicants are asked it far more often than males. But this is not the time to start quoting the law. Just give a straight-forward answer, and try not to act offended.*)

What questions do you have? (*You could ask: What do you think are this school's weaknesses and how are they being improved? What research opportunities would I have? How is your school unique? How would you describe the typical class personality here? and so on.*)

Chapter 6

The Essay

So, your transcript is complete, the MCAT is over, and you are now completing the AMCAS application. At this point, your immediate goal is to get an interview.

As we have already noted, some applicants will be rejected immediately because their scores and grades are too low, while others are almost guaranteed interviews because of their amazing numbers. For students between these two extremes (probably most of you), nothing is stamped in concrete, and a good essay can earn an interview. On the other hand, an excellent applicant who writes a sloppy essay or a weird piece about how his parents are pressuring him into medicine may in fact be writing his own rejection letter.

Everyone has an image of "the good physician," and, fair or not, you will be measured against this image. While ambition and intellect are important, the committee is also seeking students who are compassionate, sensitive, and committed to medicine. Your essay should help the interviewers develop this image of you, and you can expect them to read your essay before the interview or immediately afterwards.

Following this chapter are actual AMCAS essays by medical students accepted at Cornell, Johns Hopkins, Yale, Harvard, Columbia, Univ. of Pennsylvania, NYU, Washington University, and other top schools. We believe these pieces will give you a feel for the creativity and self-description that infuses a successful essay, and we hope they will be a catalyst for your own creativity.

We have intentionally mixed exceptional essays with the more basic, "laundry list" works to illustrate a simple point: even applicants with mediocre essays get into top medical schools. Of course, you should try to model your essay after the best presented here. To help you, we will comment briefly on the strengths and weaknesses of representative essays.

Authorship, Proofreading, and Style

This section addresses two important points. First, the ideas and writing style should be all your own! If you have not internalized a philosophy of medicine—and developed a coherent way of expressing it—it will come out in the interview.

Second, your message is more important than your writing style, but don't make a bad impression with confusing prose and inattention to detail. Deans of Admission assume your essay was proofread by Mom, Dad, a professor, a premedical advisor, and six or seven roommates, so don't hesitate to ask someone to check at least your spelling and grammar.

Essay #1 is extremely well written. The applicant clearly communicates her ideas and convinces the reader she has thought maturely about her goals. You can bet the interviewer asked her more about her view of life and her experiences with hematology/oncology and counseling.

The writing style in Essay #19 is unique. It shouts the applicant's enthusiasm and excitement about entering medicine and enjoying life. He takes the reader on a trip to the ocean, classroom, kitchen, subway, frat house, forest, and physician's office. He does not follow another's path or force himself into the premedical mold. Rather, he presents himself as a naturalist, idealist, and romantic.

If the writer of Essay #2 had not been accepted to medical school, she could have made a living as a book or movie critic. The beginning of the essay conjures vivid images of the doctor and disease, and we are left feeling that the applicant is the humanitarian. In fact, we feel she is talking about herself when she writes, "through close reading, the author's philosophy of life can be discovered." Not only does she recognize the value of the liberal arts education, she *personally* shares how she views medicine.

The best essays catch the reader's attention with an opening sentence that grabs the reader, draws him into the piece, and ties together the rest of the work. In journalism, it's called a "good lead." Examples include

Essay #45— "If you don't get paid, why the Hell do you work here?"

Essay #27— "A successful and effective physician must possess two essential qualities—a thirst for knowledge, and a deep motivation to aid his fellow man."

Essay #33— "What kind of person would be insane enough to spend half of his life studying for a job which requires twelve hour work days, no vacations, and interminable patience— in other words total dedication?"

Essay #41— "**Praeludium**. In the beginning there was dissonance."

A good lead puts readers on your side and makes them want to read more. It also makes your essay memorable.

Rather than being a hodgepodge of thoughts and achievements, your essay should also have a central theme or motif to bridge experiences, concepts, and extracurricular activities. The author of Essay #8 uses "communication" to discuss nature, philosophy of medicine, and life experiences. With society criticizing medical schools for producing impersonal robots, a poet who communicates well will stand out from the crowd.

In contrast, Essay #20 exemplifies a subtle mistake in many essays: Applicants begin their essay with an interesting concept, question, or idea, only to stray from the central theme when listing personal achievements. As a result, the body of this essay does not clearly support the lead or the conclusions. If at all possible, list your accomplishments elsewhere in the application, or have them described in your letters of recommendation. Use the essay for more personal communication.

Once you've written your final draft, there are only a few conventional standards to follow when typing your essay. Most important, be neat! Check that there are no visible corrections or spelling mistakes. This may seem obvious, but we were shocked at the number of typographical errors. Normally, applicants use a word processor or pay to have the essay professionally typed.

The length of the essay is variable. Of the essays we reviewed, some were short, such as Essay #11 with fewer than 200 words and Essay #45 with fewer than 400 words. At the other extreme, Essay #41 exceeded 1,500 words on one page. A successful essay does not have to fill the entire page with print. It's better to express your feelings and drives succinctly. (*Brevity is the soul of wit.*—Thoreau)

There is also no consistency among essays as regards margins, spacing, paragraphing, or print type. At the bottom of Essays #39 and #46, the applicants typed and signed their names. This adds a personal touch and authenticity, and may be appropriate for some.

In sum, the successful essay comes in all shapes and sizes, but its appearance and style is not nearly as important as its message.

Conservative and Safe

A conservative and safe essay can still succeed. The author of Essay #21 recognizes that many of the people who will be reading his essay are academic physicians. Saying that he eventually wants "to work in a university affiliated hospital, and to be involved in clinically related research, while maintaining patient contact" is exactly what they want to hear. He stresses he is excited about the field of medicine and believes he will enjoy caring for the sick. He mirrors his reader.

Having stressed the "correct" reasons for entering medicine, he then fills the essay with information and details which are probably interesting to the researcher and impressive to the layman—but they add little (good or bad) to the image of the applicant as a person. Early in his career, this student apparently decided to follow the Hippocratic Oath: *Primum non nocere* ("Above all, do no harm").

Often, the committee member is looking for students with a sense of balance between humanities and sciences, course work and athletics, work and fun. As an undergraduate, the applicant in Essay #26 balanced "a full dose of the humanities *and* a strong foundation in the physical sciences"—he majored in both physics and English. The woman in Essay #42 shares, "I also enjoy both listening to and performing music and hope to strike a rewarding balance between personal and professional creativity." In Essay #17, no one could question the applicant's research background. He has published two papers and four abstracts—well above the norm. Further, his proficiency in science is balanced by his artistic talent, national tours, and Broadway performances.

Again, we stress that medical schools are not seeking obsessive, compulsive students willing to lock themselves up in a lab for days. Rather, the admissions committee looks for the well-rounded applicant.

The student in Essay #5 conservatively plays the premedical game well: she worked with disadvantaged children, balanced science studies with humanities courses, conducted research at prestigious places, and gained clinical experience. She does not directly say she is a "nice" person with "nice" qualities. Instead, she compliments physicians as caring, dedicated, and intelligent. Her essay probably gave a nice boost to the ego of the reader, as well as subtly implying that she shares these attributes. This indirect method is successful.

Creative Vs. Weird

A creative essay captures the reader's attention with humor or a startling oddness. Since an interviewer reads dozens of essays in one sitting, you want your essay to be remembered—but it must be remembered in a positive way.

Effectively using dialogue, the author of Essay #9 shows he has thought about his goals in clinical medicine and at the laboratory bench. He is inquisitive and motivated, and he realizes there's more to life than straight A's.

Essay #41 won't be forgotten. Written as a piece of music, the paragraphs are divided into "Praeludium," "Allegro ma non troppo," "Andante," "Adagio," and "Allegro con spirito." Our only comment on this essay echoes what the King of Austria told Mozart after a great performance: "This opera has too many notes."

In your effort to be original, do not come across as being weird or eccentric. Skirting the bizarre, Essay #36 states: "The stories that most appeal to me are of individuals alienated from, or cast into, an alien society, struggling to assert their independence and individuality. By suspending my disbelief, I can partake in the struggle of the fictional characters and feel their victories and defeats." The applicant recognizes that he is challenging psychological norms and continues, "I am careful, however, not to confuse my love of adventure and fantasy with my reasons for wanting to be a physician." However, we wonder whether he would have been so bold if he knew that admissions committees often ask psychiatrists to interview applicants who write anything unusual in their essays. Take heed.

Apologetic, Egotistical, Doubtful, or Boring

As a rule, don't use the essay to apologize for a low grade or a less than perfect MCAT score, as in #11 or #39. Nobody is perfect, and admissions committees don't want a litany of excuses. They're looking for good reasons to accept you, not trivial reasons to weed you out. Instead, use the space to present positive information about yourself.

Essay #16 comes across as somewhat egotistical, and it exemplifies what *not* to write. There's no question that he has expertise in the lab, and his knowledge of AIDS makes him an attractive candidate. But a commitment to patients should be foremost— and in the first paragraph, not the last line. He should have emphasized his concern in a positive way, not the negative way of "I will not divorce myself from patient care." He constantly places himself first, and though that may be a characteristic of many ambitious people, it doesn't make for a sympathetic essay. He expresses "realistic concerns for the safety of myself" and anxiety about the AIDS virus appearing in his own low-risk group. He says his greatest satisfaction is in the laboratory—before he mentions the plight of the AIDS patient. Twice he boasts about receiving strong recommendations and being the only student approved to enter his laboratory.

Obviously, this applicant has a lot going for him, but his essay is a real turn-off. With a little perspective—that is, put yourself in the *reader's* shoes—you can appear talented and positive without being arrogant. Allow your credentials to speak for themselves.

One essay we reviewed made a mistake by ending, "The school that accepts me will receive an excited student who will prove to the board of admissions that they did not make a mistake." Although the student wants to leave the committee with the message that he is "excited" about medicine, the reader instead is left wondering why it would be a "mistake" to admit him. What does the applicant feel he has to "prove to the board of admissions" after the fact? Maybe if your entire application is strong, the question is irrelevant, but if there's a weakness in your application, leave it alone.

A mature, appropriate sense of humor never hurts. In Essay #29, the author stresses how his in-depth knowledge of biological sciences and microbiology will be useful when studying "*Neisseria gonnorhoae*." Whether intentional or not, it's a funny prediction. On the other hand, Essay #24 is amusing in the way the author sets the reader up by mentioning impressive accomplishments achieved in the past and possibly reached in the future. He then matter-of-factly presents unachievable personal goals. Amuse the reader and you will be remembered.

Why a Physician?

Why you decided to become a doctor is a common essay theme. Some students always knew they wanted to be physicians, in the same way children decide they want to be a fireman, a teacher, or President of the United States. The applicant of Essay #39 states that she knew as a child she would be a physician when she grew up, and she discusses how her decision was logically reaffirmed over the years.

However, every physician did not choose medicine as a kid playing with a toy stethoscope. Essay #34 typifies how most students shape their goals. This applicant mentions how his experiences as an E.M.T. on an ambulance crew and rescue squad were "invaluable training for a career in medicine." Some students, on the other hand, discuss the influence of literature on their decision to pursue medicine. In Essay #3, the student is inspired by Doctor Dolittle and Charles Darwin, while the author of Essay #2 is influenced by a character in *The Plague*.

Professional paths are best decided with maturity and insight. The applicant of Essay #22 began bird-watching in college, had a gut feeling he would enjoy medicine, and tested his interest with clinical, research, and volunteer experiences. He has a good feeling for what is ahead of him: "The science may interest me, the diagnoses may challenge me, but it will be that personal involvement with the patient that will make the most difference to me and keep me going through the hardest parts."

Translating Research Into Clinical Practice

In general, the most prestigious medical schools emphasize basic research. While only a handful of students actually pursue academic medicine, almost all successful applicants have at least token laboratory experience.

In your essay, you may choose to mention what you did, where you worked, and with whom. In any case, you will want to stress how much you enjoy research (embellish if necessary).

For example, in Essay #33 the student recalls "an incredible high" when his first scientific paper was published. The student in Essay #40 states, "In the long run though, I would like to be a physician who researches medicine on a 'basic science' level and, at the same time, translates advances in scientific theory into clinical practice." Likewise, the applicant in Essay #42 concludes, "I would therefore gain satisfaction from involvement in both the research aspect of medicine and its practical applications in patient care."

Don't panic if you haven't done lab work. You can still mention your dream of pursuing (time permitting) the Nobel Prize in Medicine. And if you aren't convincing, remember that research experience is neither required nor expected at less competitive institutions. Some applicants can get accepted without ever spending a weekend with a pipette, flask, or bunsen burner.

If you really enjoy research, consider the M.D.-Ph.D. programs listed at the end of Chapter 5. If selected, you receive a nice stipend, and your education is completely paid for (Mom and Dad will love that). When applying to an intensive joint program like an M.D.-Ph.D., be sure your essay shows balance. Don't discuss research for 99% of the essay, and then give one line to medicine. Remember that biomedical research, treating patients, and teaching are three equally important aspects of academic medicine. Essays #10 and #17 make this point well. Nonetheless, the author of Essay #11 is an M.D.-Ph.D. applicant, and his essay addressed only academics (and briefly), but worked.

Meeting the Physician Shortage

Most medical schools actively recruit qualified minority students who express an interest in serving segments of the population that don't have access to excellent medical care.

In Essay #6, the applicant, a Mexican-American, has considered practicing in a needy Latin American country. He expresses altruistic motives, and he shows scientific aptitude with his authorship on a published paper.

The student in Essay #38 had his interest in medicine sparked after participating in the American Foundation for Negro Affairs Program. Later, he worked in a hematology department testing for sickle cell anemia, a common blood disorder among blacks.

The applicant in Essay #29 states, "My ethnic background has been a contributing factor in my prospective plans after medical school. I would like to work in a physician shortage area where my Puerto Rican background will be helpful in dealing with other Hispanic minorities." She believes it is her "duty in life" to care for others. Essay #43 was also written by a Hispanic who has worked with the poor.

Women as a group are underrepresented in medicine. Since medicine has been a male-dominated profession, the female doctor sometimes confronts sexist attitudes. The woman in Essay #32 states, "Medicine was a serious consideration but due to the conservative attitude of my parents and Switzerland, the idea of a woman in medicine was not well supported." More alarming than parental pressures are the many female applicants who tell the story of a male doctor who asked during the interview, "Won't your career be ruined when you have a family?" (But remember, he may only have been trying to rattle them.)

The applicant in Essay #10 has insight into the concerns of

many admissions officers about the role of women in medicine. She has chosen to confront sexism by describing a successful woman/physician/scientist who also has a happy family life. The applicant feels she can balance her profession and personal life, and she addresses the issue up front.

Older students often have gained skills and knowledge in fields that might further medicine. One applicant we know attended Bible college and wants to become a missionary doctor. The applicant in Essay #46 pursued a Ph.D. in psychobiology. We also know students who first worked as investment bankers, teachers, scientists, police officers, and even medical school professors before beginning medical school.

Admissions committees do not expect applicants to know for certain the field of practice they will enter. However, if you think you want to work in an under-served region or less-popular specialty, say so. The minority student in Essay #7 wants to improve health care for the indigent and the elderly. His interests in academic medicine and public health are admirable, because they are areas of medicine criticized for lacking dedicated physicians. He acknowledges that he has benefited from special opportunities made available to him, and now he says he's eager to use his background to help society. This applicant also improved his chances for admission by participating in a summer program at his first-choice medical school while applying.

Good medical care is also lacking in many rural areas, where the applicant in Essay #12 wants to practice. She describes how her goals developed and how her interests are consistent with her goals. With admissions committees knowledgeable about the health problems facing rural areas, they would be hesitant to toss this application into a rejection pile.

Other areas of physician shortage include primary care, public policy, armed forces, pediatrics, oncology, and geriatrics. Essays #26, #27, #29, and #34 express interest in these fields of practice.

Stamina

In the past, endurance was extremely important for medical school admission, and a physical handicap would completely eliminate a person's chances for admission. Today, although most of our classmates are in excellent physical shape, some have speech, vision, or other disabilities.

Athletic involvement is a measure of physical stamina—and, presumably, your ability to withstand long nights in the emergency room. Essays #24, #32, and #44 all describe athletic exploits that indicate physical strength and a well-rounded person.

Mental stamina is equally important, and the admissions committee often respects a tough academic major. This probably accounts for engineers having such good luck with admissions. Essays #31, #35, and #38 were written by engineers. The applicant of Essay #38 already applied his skills and developed various prosthetics. And don't forget other challenging undergraduate majors, as in Essay #40. Statistically, economics majors fare well, too.

In addition to physical stamina and academic rigors, mental outlook is an important indicator used by the admissions committee to assess an applicant's fitness for medicine. In Essay #33, the student shares how asthma has influenced his life and decision to become a physician. The applicant in Essay #30 mentions his father's battle with schizophrenia and how the son matured because of the tragedy. In Essay #42, because the applicant witnessed the death of family members, she felt compelled to do her part to integrate modern science with medicine. Similarly, the applicant in Essay #48 was motivated to pursue medicine after helplessly watching a person die.

Witnessing illnesses and deaths are powerful influences. How you cope with tragedy is very much a part of the everyday life of a doctor.

Admissions committees will gain a sense of how you deal with the stresses inherent in medicine by how you respond to other types of adversity or pressures (as in the interview). The applicant in Essay #13 does not falter after a negative college event, but turns it into a positive, maturing, and motivating experience. (As a side note, just because the AMCAS application states that the applicant needs to explain any disciplinary action during college, don't assume you should devote the whole page to details. It's better to mention what you learned or how the adversity has helped direct you.)

The M.D. Family

Sons and daughters of physicians pervade the medical school class. Historically, this is consistent with the Hippocratic Oath, which instructs the doctor "to regard his offspring as equal . . . and to teach them this art—if they desire to learn it."

Moreover, doctor's kids know what they're getting into. They know about the stress and its toll on the family. Children of physicians have a more realistic view of medicine, its practice, its demands, and its rewards.

Essays #18, #25, #26, #37, #44 were written by children of physicians.

Name-Dropping

If you work for someone you know and respect, chances are he or she has many other friends as well. Essays #10, #28, #33, #42 describe by name their role models.

The physician in the first essay, for example, was known and liked at many of the medical schools to which the student applied. The applicant told us that once she learned that the interviewer and she had a mutual friend, she relaxed and did much better in the interview. It's easier to impress someone who already has a good reason to like you.

Likewise, the applicant in Essay #32 says her husband is at Cornell Medical School. Having a spouse at a particular medical school may help gain the applicant an interview. Medical students often write letters on behalf of their spouses, boyfriends, or girlfriends. With a strong applicant, a letter of support may convince an admissions committee that the student will matriculate if offered an acceptance letter. The alternative is a medical student who might transfer to another medical school later to join his or her spouse. Admissions committees dislike losing students to other schools and feel guilty about breaking up a family or romance.

The point is, if you have an inside connection, make it known to the committee.

Besides using personal contacts, some applicants will actually name the medical school they want to attend in their AMCAS essay. We think this is a very risky tactic, but the applicant in Essay #46 knows where she wants to go: "I have chosen the Cornell Program due to its newly established PET facility as well as its exceptional reputation in the neurosciences."

We caution that name-dropping may limit your options. Presumably, the candidate in Essay #15 planned to attend Buffalo, Baylor, or Cornell. Experience and the contacts she made working at these schools gives her an edge, but unless you are totally set on attending a particular school, don't name-drop. Medical schools won't want to send an acceptance letter to someone they'll probably lose to another school. Remember, you must convince each medical school that it is among your top choices.

A personal story from Daniel: Many interviewers will ask, "What schools have you interviewed with?" Well, one school that interviewed me was SUNY Buffalo, where the interviewer asked me point-blank which school was my first choice and why. I was tempted to lie and say Buffalo, but I straddled the fence. "I am very interested in Buffalo," I replied, "but I would consider Cornell if I were to have a choice." After a while, he let me change the subject.

At the end of the hour, he studied my application again while he made me wait for what seemed like eternity. He then closed my file, tossed my application onto his desk, and said, "Mr. Jones, I do not think you're going to be coming here."

I really blew it! I thought. I felt I had nothing to lose, so I challenged him. "What do you mean?" He explained that he thought I'd get into Cornell with no problem. He seemed to overlook that I had not yet interviewed there—a fact foremost in *my* mind. I reminded him that I liked the people I had met at Buffalo, that I thought the tuition was reasonable, and that I didn't mind the weather. In the end, Buffalo did accept me, but the doctor was right. I got into Cornell.

The lesson: doctors aren't stupid, and the interviewer will know you're lying—or at least being insincere—if you say you're dying to go to Podunk Medical School instead of Yale. So don't lie!

A Word of Warning

As you read the essays that follow, you might be tempted to highlight good lines and incorporate them verbatim into your own essay. Some students, unfortunately, might even want to swipe the whole piece and just "change it around a little."

We hope you realize how incredibly dumb that would be. Most admissions officers have read this book and these essays, and they would never admit a plagiarist. Any doubts about your integrity will destroy your application and your reputation.

About the Essays

When you sit down to write your personal statement, we hope you'll use the essays as a catalyst to your creativity. As you read them, we think you'll be relieved to learn how broad the stylistic range is and how diverse the "acceptable" topics are.

The essays should also assist you as you consider your motivations for entering medicine and try to explain them. We cannot stress enough how important it is to be able to articulate your goals during the interview.

Each essay is reprinted exactly as it was written on the application. We have not corrected grammar, punctuation, or spelling errors. But note that rarely would such correction be necessary. Occasionally, we have changed proper names and locations to guarantee anonymity.

Finally, we would again like to express our gratitude to the generous young doctors who allowed us to reprint their essays.

Fifty
Successful
AMCAS
Essays

Essay #1

My mother has told me that as a child my favorite question was "how come?" Rarely content with a simple explanation, I seemed constantly to have pushed my parents to give me more details about the way the world worked. This inquisitiveness, while sometimes the subject of affectionate joking, was always encouraged, even when answers were not available. I learned to value the explorative process as much as any "answer" found, and spent much of my free time discovering meadows and brooks, building imaginary civilizations, or immersing myself in a book. My parents are both English professors, and their love of the humanities has always been a vital part of my life. Although my exposure to the sciences at home was limited, I avidly pursued any outside opportunities to learn about the scientific world, and during my high school years the excitement of scientific discovery began to surpass any previous intellectual experiences I had had. Continuing with the humanities, I began to discover that for me novels and music were a luxury, offering pleasure and release. The happiness I derived from them did not have to be forsaken, but could be continued while I pursued a career in science.

Entering Wesleyan University, I thought I would major in Biology while simultaneously exploring as many other fields as possible, but my actual career goals were still hazy. I had previously acquired a taste for scholarship when I worked at Williams College as an archival assistant, but the somewhat solitary nature of the work had lead me to question my desire for a career devoted exclusively to research. During my first two years at Wesleyan, I took several laboratory corses, and found that although they were extremely time consuming, I was excited by the way classroom concepts came alive in the laboratory. Towards the end of my sophomore year a possible career in medicine first became a reality for me. Much that I valued seemed to be present within this field: the opportunity to acquire scientific knowledge, to do research, and to work with and help people. Seeking summer work that would give me the opportunity to explore medicine and medical research, I was fortunate enough to obtain a position in the Department of Hematology/Oncology at UCLA Hospital, with Dr. Martin Cline.

I am still awed by what occurred that summer. At nineteen, I walked into one of the most exciting and meaningful sectors of research in the country. The discoveries that were made while I worked in Dr. Cline's lab were extraordinary, and because I was an integral part of the functioning lab, I felt like an explorer myself. Since part of my responsibility involved getting cancer samples from the hospital every day, I also spent some time in the operating room and a lot of time in pathology. The exposure to clinical and surgical work was as valuable and stimulating as the research. The work was fascinating, the challenge a bit frightening, but I soon felt at ease in both lab and hospital. All that I had learned seemed to come miraculously together that summer.

The doctors I worked for became my mentors. I had not previously realized that one could be both a clinician and a research scientist, and while I sensed that research alone would not fulfill my needs, I still felt a desire to explore this option further. I looked forward to the research I had arranged to do at Wesleyan on my return. At the same time, however, I wanted more experience working directly with people, and when I went back to school in the fall, I trained to be a "listener" for 8 to 8, a student-run counseling service.

My junior year has been thoroughly enriched by my research and counseling experiences. The 8 to 8 training process was invaluable. Through it I learned a lot about myself—my attributes, faults, and values—and about human psychology. Working for the counseling service has strengthed considerably my conviction that medicine is, for me, an ideal vocation, one that would allow me to unite my scientific interests with the personal satisfaction I gain from helping and working with people. The research I am conducting at Wesleyan has been equally fulfilling. As my research experience has grown, my thought processes have slowly begun to change. Designing experiments, I have realized, requires foresight and a thorough integration of many concepts learned in the classroom, abilities I think are important for a doctor to possess, and that I hope I can continue to develop. This summer, at Brigham and Women's Hospital, I will again be doing research, and look forward to exploring still further the world of the laboratory.

My research experiences have been wonderfully rewarding, and I hope to continue laboratory work both through and after medical school. Clinical practice, however, is fundamentally more important to me, because it brings together my interest in people and my scientific and humanitarian ideals. I feel thoroughly committed to a career in medicine and only hope that I am able to give the profession as much as I think it can give to me.

Essay #2

The narrator and hero of Albert Camus' novel, *The Plague*, is a doctor named Bernard Rieux. Amidst the horror of the plague which grips his city, the bureaucratic ineptitude, the religious fanaticism embraced by one character and the bleak existentialism presented by another, Dr. Rieux emerges as an advocate for the strength of human will and love. While the epidemic strikes people dead at random, rendering the efforts of medical science impotent, Rieux refuses to succumb to the belief that life is meaningless and tirelessly fights the plague with what little means he has. Romantic as this scenario sounds, Camus presents it objectively, and the novel's power lies in its almost journalistic reality.

When I read *The Plague* in high school, I was greatly drawn to the characteer of Rieux because of his humanism and because in the face of the epidemic he as a doctor was the only one who could actively do anything, though not much, to combat the disaster. The impotence which he felt against the plague is what all people must feel against any disease, although in many cases medicine can help a great deal. I had some contact with disease and injury while volunteering at a children's hospital in Cleveland. The patients ranged in age from two to twenty, and I visited them in their rooms, played games with or read to them, or just talked. I was glad to be able to give some emotional aid, but I felt powerless to change their condition. The dynamic power of medical science seemed very appealing to me during that experience.

However, as Camus illustrates through Dr. Rieux, being a physician involves more than scientific knowledge and its application. True sympathy—the ability to place oneself in the position of another—is what Rieux achieves and is what makes him a great doctor. I feel that studying literature is one of the best means of expanding one's sympathy. Not only does reading literature require an immersion in the emotional world of the characters, but through close reading, the author's philosophy of life can be discovered. This interpretation is what makes literature so challenging; the ideas are often not explicitly defined. I decided to major in English because I wanted an opportunity to study literature in depth and be able to discuss it with classmates and professors.

In addition to literature, I have taken many history courses, which I feel are equally as important to a liberal arts education. Knowing history helps one to place current social issues in perspective. Most of the history courses I have taken touched upon issues relevant to medicine and society. In an English history course, for example, I read about physicians in the eighteenth century who stole corpses from the gallows for anatomical dissection, because the supply of cadavers for research was strictly controlled by the government. The outrage of witnesses to this practice is paralleled by current public concern about the ethics of medical research, especially in the field of genetics. In my American history courses we covered topics ranging from the unrecognized outbreaks of malaria and typhus which killed many of the first settlers at Jamestown, to the establishment of Medicare under Lyndon Johnson. Studying history makes one aware of the tremendous advances in medical science, and also of the continuity of human attitudes towards medicine.

My own belief that humanism is vital to being a physician was reinforced during the summer I spent working in the Euclid Clinic. I helped patients settle their accounts and fill out insurance forms, so I had a great deal of patient contact. Most of the patients I saw had come directly from a doctor's office, and many of them wanted to talk about their visit. A frequent complaint which I heard was that their doctors rarely took time to listen to questions and worries, or give explanations and reassurance. The patients felt a need to tell someone about their illness or injury, and I spent a lot of time listening. My experience that summer left me with the feeling that although scientific skill may be the most important quality in a doctor, it is not the only necessary quality.

Essay #3

I want to become a physician to heal people and to further my study of man as both creative thinker and purely biological animal. I think I've always been sensitive to the needs of others, and my experiences of the past few years have indicated to me that as a medical doctor I can make the progressive social contribution that is one of my life goals.

As a child I was preoccupied with things biological. I remember digging patiently among ants in their tunnels and trying to locate the eggs, capturing different bees from flowers, attempting to raise bird chicks fallen from their nests, and poring over slides of my blood and hair with a small microscope. Once I learned what the word meant I fancied myself a naturalist, and took great pleasure in the observations I made in the woods and marsh near our home. My favorite childhood books were Hugh Lofting's *Doctor Dolittle* series and Daniel Defoe's *Robinson Crusoe*. Later I read about Charles Darwin and John J. Audubon.

In high school I excelled in science subjects and was placed in advanced courses; I also concentrated on English and foreign languages. There was time for playing on the soccer team, practicing the cello, and writing for the school and community newspapers. I became more aware of chronic social problems, and passionately so. I took the AP courses in history and studied the evolution of man's endeavors to solve those problems. I discovered distinctions between various interpretations of objective history and visions of the future. I realized that while advances in technology were necessary for progress, their proper application was an equally important and complex issue. Technical advances in medicine, for example, are in themselves amazing but their utility is subject to ethical and economic considerations.

I viewed college as an opportunity for experimentation as well as for the pursuit of my established interests. I became interested in health care specifically while volunteering in the local Cerebral Palsy clinic. Our group worked primarily with young people in a weekly swim/gym program. I met on a regular basis with two boys who shared an uneasy friendship and were eager for attention from an adult. Once established, our relationship was a source of pleasure for me as well as for them. Hospital work in later years confirmed my positive attitude towards dealing with sick and handicapped people. Though I took premedical courses at Williams College, I was not intensely career-oriented. I wanted a broad education and chose history as its foundation. For my junior year I sought an experience outside the "ivory tower" of Williams. I attended the London School of Economics & Political Science, whose highly specialized curriculum complemented my more diverse program at home. Stimulated by the emphasis on independent work, I immersed myself in the study of modern history.

Following graduation from Williams I received a grant to serve as field assistant with a research team studying the physiology of the Black Rhinoceros in Kenya under the auspices of Harvard and Nairobi Universities. We worked with the Kenyan Game Dept. in moving the rare animals from highly poached areas to safer ones. Our group had access to the temporarily captive rhinos in order to record physiological data relevant to thermoregulation studies.

The rhino project ended in Sept. '80 but I stayed in Kenya to work with an ecologist doing a study of the carrying capacity for elephants in Meru National Park. When herds are confined to limited areas, their feeding destroys the vegetation quickly, and an aspect of large game management is determining the population a park can support. For a rapidly growing nation like Kenya, the problem is real; people are hungry and have little sympathy for animals that leave the parks to eat their crops. Actually I found the human side of the issue to be crucial; as both our needs and technology grow, so does our potential environmental impact. Development programs including a rational allocation of resources have become necessary to provide for both the "manmade" and "natural" worlds.

Medical care is one especially important part of the development strategy I'm referring to and is the focus of my interest. All through Kenya, Sudan, and Egypt I was amazed at the success of medical clinics that have, in fighting infectious disease, helped to raise birth and survival rates and life expectancies—but not necessarily the quality of life! More children survive into adulthood only to suffer from chronic malnutrition. Yet impoverished parents often rely on their children for security and disregard government urgings to limit family size. I feel that lay health education is an important adjunct to medical care programs.

The two years I spent in Africa and the Middle East experiencing vastly different cultures and living conditions have given me a new perspective here at home. I also gained confidence from dealing with accidents and other difficult situations that I hadn't encountered in school. I feel strongly that I have the potential for personal as well as professional growth in the study and practice of medicine.

Essay #4

At the age of six I started studying insects under my magnifying glass and by the time I was ten, I had already detonated my first explosive with the help of a Mr. Wizard chemistry kit. These are just the first entries in my scientific resume. In high school I became more serious, studying the areas of electronics and meteorology at the Talcott Mountain Science Center in Avon, Connecticut, and holographic photography at the Weizmann Institute of Science in Israel. Once in college, I became a biology teaching assistant and a physics tutor in addition to my regular schedule of science courses. There was rarely a time when I was not involved in some type of science-related activity. More recently, however, I have discovered that there is another world outside the scientific establishment: one that has made me aware of my inner strengths, my capacity to handle responsibility, and my sensitivity towards other people.

It was in the mountains of Wyoming where I learned the true meaning of challenge. As part of a two-week winter camping and survival course taught by the National Outdoor Leadership School (NOLS), I camped out in temperatures of twenty-seven degrees below zero, cross-country skied with a seventy pound pack, and climbed to altitudes that could not sustain vegetation. Survival, not the allurement of the alpine environment, was my only thought. It was not until I had time to reflect upon my adventures that I realized what it meant to persevere. I knew I could apply those characteristics of determination, will, and desire to any future situation.

My participation in an American Youth Hostel (AYH) leadership training course is where I learned the skills of leadership and responsibility. Here, for the first time, I was responsible for the welfare of others as I conducted a group bicycle tour across Ohio. After nine days of pedaling through the farmlands of Pandora, replacing the broken spokes of Fuji bicycles and settling the common arguments among my companion bikers, i.e., when to eat, whose turn it was to clean up, and how to spend group funds, I understood what responsibility entailed. It was more than directing a group towards a destination. It was listening to their problems and helping each one see different viewpoints. It was consoling a forty-five year-old woman when her rear wheel was hopelessly bent, and it was helping a fellow college student whip up a late dinner for an unruly group.

While the NOLS and AYH programs are just two short experiences in my life, what I took from them has enabled me to see how important people are in my future. I know now that I enjoy working with all types of people, that I will not shy away from difficult problems, and that I have the skills and temperament to handle various situations. This knowledge, coupled with my interest in science, has inspired me to seek a career that combines humanism with scientific expertise.

This summer I have accepted a position in the Hartford Hospital Student Fellowship Program where I am involved in pulmonary function testing under the supervision of Dr. Arthur DeGraff. This program has enabled me to witness certain clinical procedures which have confirmed what I always felt inherent in the medical profession: that physicians are not just scientists but have a concern for other people, are able to persevere in difficult situations, and accept responsibility in life and death matters. While there is a great physical difference between the mountains of Wyoming and the corridors of Hartford Hospital, both have given me a new insight into myself and the medical profession. I now hope to study medicine and become the type of physician who is as comfortable with a stethoscope as he is with a patient's complaint.

Essay #5

I would like to share a number of personal experiences that contributed to my decision to become a physician.

I first became interested in science in high school when an extremely talented teacher introduced me to the study of biology. Although the course was only an introductory one, this teacher went far beyond the standard curriculum. Not only did the class dissect frogs, grasshoppers, and worms, but it also proceeded under his direction to dissect cow eyes, and the brains and hearts of sheep. As the course progressed, the teacher's enthusiasm for his subject made me, in turn, eager to learn more. Thus my introduction to science at the high school level was very positive, and I looked forward to pursuing a science-related career.

Another high school experience was also to prove instrumental in my future career choice. I was involved in a program in which students volunteered at Suffolk Development Center, a state-run mental institution in Melville, New York. Each volunteer was assigned to one patient on a regular basis. My charge, Joey, was a nineteen-year-old boy, who was blind, mentally retarded, and crippled. Quite frankly, the experience at first made me uncomfortable—I had never before been exposed to such severely handicapped people—but my initial feeling subsided as I became more involved with helping Joey perform simple tasks which, for him, were major accomplishments. This experience made me sensitive to the need to provide facilities for those whose health is mentally or physically impaired, and taught me that patience, care, and determination are needed to help such people. It was at this time that I began to focus on a career in medicine.

Because I was aware that the practice of medicine involved not only scientific principles, but a real understanding of the human condition, I sought in college to place my interest in science within a broad humanist perspective. I particularly enjoyed my Classics courses, and as for my science courses, it was Electron Microscopy that made the deepest impression on me. Here I was able to view in fine detail the complexity of cells and tissues. This course also provided me with an opportunity to work independently—preparing tissue, examining it under the microscope, and analyzing the various histological structures.

During my college years, I was able to observe the practical application of scientific knowledge. For example, I spent the month of January of my sophomore year in the Human Genetics Department of the Yale University School of Medicine. I attended medical school genetics classes, as well as various medical conferences. Most important, however, under the direction of Dr. Xandra O. Breakfield, I engaged in an independent research project involving the bloodstream activity of the enzyme dopamine-B-hydroxylase and its possible basis of genetic inheritance. Although the results of the project were inconclusive, the experience proved to be very helpful to me, because it gave me an understanding of how scientific research can be used to study clinical problems.

My understanding of the field of medicine was enhanced during the following summer when, as a student intern, I was able to observe the activities of physicians in various specialties at Booth Memorial Hospital in Flushing, New York. These specialties included General Surgery, Pathology, Pediatrics, Endocrinology, and Radiology. I also spent time in the Emergency Room, the Clinic, and the Intensive Care Unit. This experience enabled me to appreciate the role of the doctor in both a hospital setting and private practice. In addition, my internship gave me an introduction to the advanced technology used in modern hospitals, and it also allowed me to observe firsthand the more intangible components of the practice of the art of medicine: the care, compassion, and dedication that these professionals demonstrated.

Because my experience at Booth was so valuable, I wanted to use the summer of 1983 to add to my knowledge of the medical field. I applied, therefore, to the Sarah Lawrence Program for Pre-Medical Students at Lawrence Hospital in Bronxville, New York, and I have been accepted. This program attempts to provide an overview of the medical experience while focusing on the students' personal interests. I look forward, in particular, to spending time in Emergency Medicine, Endocrinology, and Pathology.

My various experiences in high school and college have shown me that the field of medicine demands intelligence, integrity, compassion, and commitment, and I believe that my personal attributes will enable me to make a positive contribution to the profession.

Essay #6

Throughout my young life, I have constantly strived to answer the questions presented before me. Some have been easy—"What is the square root of 9,801?" (99). Others have not been quite so simple—"What do you want to be when you grow up? Why?" My first science courses in the 7th grade stimulated my interest in the medical profession. Before long, I had even selected a speciality: neurosurgery.

Although I have almost always had set goals, I have not been afraid to challenge them. From my sophomore year through my high school graduation, I worked as a typist/computer programmer (15-20 hr/wk, five d/wk) in a small music stand business. This job not only allowed me to improve my dexterity, but also to contribute to my family's strained budget; thus I tasted my first responsibility in the real world. Although I briefly considered a career in computers, I soon realized that I would gain little sense of contribution to other people.

During my first two years in college I worked as an attendant (20 hr/wk) at a local video arcade. Constant interaction with customers made my employment there well worthwhile.

The summer following my sophomore year, I found a job as a lab assistant (30 hr/wk, 1½ mos) in the neuroresearch center of the VA Hospital in Palo Alto, CA. At first I worked as a simple lab technician. Before long, however, my supervisor became convinced that I had the potential to do more, and I was taught to inject rats and to perform a simple surgical maneuver—crush a nerve in the leg and sew the surrounding muscles and skin back together. Although I worked in this lab for a relatively short time, the exposure piqued my interest in the field of research, an option I am currently considering quite seriously.

Acting on this new-found interest in research, I took on a job in the psychobiology labs on Berkeley campus (10-15 hrs/wk, 5 d/wk 1st sem; 5 h/wk, 3 d/wk 2nd and 3rd sems, as projects became less demanding). I wrote two reports while receiving academic credit, describing how a component of long-term memory in rats could be affected by certain drugs. In these papers I designed several original statistical analyses and, in a recently published paper of which I was a co-author, we showed for the first time that long-term memory could be used in a manner not previously considered. Here I was able to interact with professionals as I gained a much more in-depth, rewarding exposure to life in the labs.

In addition to volunteering my time in the labs, I have supported myself by typing an organic chemistry textbook (10-20 h/wk, 5 d/wk; full-time during the summers). This job has been particularly rewarding, as the author allowed me to start editing the book from a student's point of view. My goal has been to present organic chemistry to future students in a clearer and more interesting fashion than it was presented to me.

Although I have enjoyed the challenge of medical research and studies, I have gained increasing satisfaction from contributing my services to others. For the past three years, I have participated in our campus "Buddy" orientation program. Perhaps my greatest satisfaction came when one particular "buddy" (who had been out of school for almost eight years) came to me for help. At first, the shock of university life seemed to be pushing her on the verge of a nervous breakdown, but as I continued to volunteer countless hours of both tutoring (something I have always enjoyed doing) and moral support, she finally began to calm down, and now performs at or near the top of her classes. There may be nothing on this earth more rewarding than helping someone else realize his or her potential!

Having repeatedly reaffirmed my career choice as a physician and/or medical researcher, I realized that I had virtually no experience helping actual patients. Consequently, I started working this February in the ever-busy trauma center at San Francisco General. Before long I found myself working every Friday night from 11 p.m. to 4 a.m., helping physicians and nurses complete a variety of tasks (lab-runs, guerney sheet-changes, etc.). More important, however, my primary role has been to provide moral support to and respond to the needs of often-confused and frightened patients. I have even been able to use my Spanish-speaking ability (acquired in part from my Mexican-American background) to help patients that did not know English. Trauma room life has been so exciting that I constantly find myself watching the physicians at work and helping them in any way possible, even by performing CPR on occasion. The satisfaction I have received in making the patients' visits as pleasant as possible, as well as in making the staff's work a little easier, has been inestimable. At four in the morning, I'm almost never ready to leave!

My biggest question now is no longer whether I want to be a doctor, but whether I want to be a specialist, as earlier planned, or a GP, where my services could be more useful, especially in needy Latin American countries. The decision may not be too difficult if my experiences keep going the way they have been!

Essay #7

The problems of our society, particularly those related to health care delivery, are numerous. Solutions to these problems will arise from individuals who have a broad view of society and the will to contribute their talents to society. I feel that I possess these qualities and can best contribute my talents to society as a physician.

It was as a junior in high school that I began to consider pursuing a career in medicine. I decided to participate in Project SOAR, a summer premedical program at Xavier. As a participant in Project SOAR, I had the opportunity to learn about medicine by speaking to students who had been accepted by medical schools. By exposing me to college-level work and successful premedical students, whose academic backgrounds were similar to my own, SOAR enhanced my confidence in my academic ability and encouraged me to pursue a career in medicine.

During my senior year in high school, I enrolled as a part-time student in the Concurrent Admissions program at Xavier, where I attended six semester hours of credit. My experiences in Project SOAR and in the Concurrent Admissions program influenced my decision to matriculate at Xavier, full-time, as a chemistry major.

Pursuing a career in medicine is a challenge that should be undertaken only by persons who have a genuine interest in health care. I have learned that I would enjoy working as a physician to improve the quality of health care in our society. My experience in the 1984 United Negro College Fund Summer Premedical Institute affirmed my interest in medicine and provided me with information about a variety of exciting medical careers. I will participate in the 1986 Summer Research Fellowship Program at the Cornell University Medical College, where my research assignment will involve nuclear medicine. Clinical exposure is also a component of the program. I look forward to the experience, since it should provide me with a better understanding of the role of research in medicine.

At Xavier I have had the opportunity to gain teaching experience. I instructed a general chemistry class, one day each week, during the fall semester of 1984, and in 1985 I taught high school students who participated in a summer chemistry program. Assisting my students in reaching their academic goals was very rewarding. Teaching was very enjoyable, because it allowed me to work with people in a meaningful way. I feel that I would enjoy practicing medicine, since it would allow me to interact with people in a similar manner.

Presently I am interested in diagnostic imaging and academic medicine. Because I am very interested in social issues, I am also considering pursuing the degree of Master of Public Health, so that I may better serve the health care delivery system.

Physicians, like other citizens, have a vested interest in the well-being of society. They should be involved not only in treating patients, but also in solving the problems of health care delivery, such as providing medical care to the indigent and the elderly. Although my career goals are not definite at this time, I feel that my background is such that I can pursue a career in any area of medicine and make a meaningful contribution to society. Moreover, my ability to work with others strengthens my conviction that medicine is my vocation. For these reasons, I believe that I can best serve society as a physician.

Essay #8

During college my closest friends and I have spent hours analyzing our personalities and determining what makes us unique. We explored what motivated our becoming good doctors and why it would make us happy, and we examined the underlying currents which influence and motivate our thoughts and actions. For me, the most visible current is communication: being able to articulate my thoughts, being able to make others experience them, being receptive to the ideas of others, and being understanding.

As a poet, I feel that in order to write meaningful poetry, one must have a clear sense of how to communicate effectively. Whenever I begin a poem, I remember the advice of my high school English teacher: "a poem should be wordless, as the flight of birds." By choosing precise words, by paying attention to the sounds of phrases sewn together, and by evoking clear images, a poem is created. It should grip and move the reader immediately just as a person, seeing a perfectly wedged V-line of Canadian geese flying overhead toward the horizon, stops, catches his breath, and reflects on the beauty that has passed. It is through poetry that I try to recapture my feelings during those wordless moments, and I try to pass them on to the reader.

My need to be a communicator extends beyond poetry. Learning foreign languages, peer counseling, student advising, tutoring, and acting are activities in which I have participated. Each activity emphasizes a particular discipline of communication. Learning foreign languages stems from my enjoyment of communicating with people of different cultures in their native languages. By speaking a language common to us both, communication barriers are bridged. A peer counseling center offers students a comfortable place to talk. By attentive listening, the counselor helps the student clarify his thoughts and feelings and explore options to his problems. Student advisors form quick, friendly rapports with the incoming freshmen. Throughout the year, the advisors offer guidance and suggest options and opportunities at college by relating their own experiences. The tutoring process centers on imparting knowledge. The tutor must motivate the student to cope with his difficulties, to overcome them, and to finally enjoy learning the subject. My involvement in acting and directing is a form of personal expression through interpretation. I draw upon my experiences and intuition to present realistic, complex portrayals.

Through foreign languages, peer counseling, student advising, tutoring, and theater, I have explored and developed my communicative abilities. It is this aspect of my personality that will be challenged by a medical career. Whenever one studies foreign languages, one learns to be receptive to a foreign culture. With a perceptive and sympathetic ear is how the peer counselor listens. A student advisor is a freshman's first friend, and a tutor becomes a trusted teacher. An actor or a director investigates the endless possibilities of presenting characters and scenes in certain viewpoints. A doctor embodies the essential characteristics of all these people. A receptive student, a patient listener, an approachable friend, an informative conveyor, and a perceptive examiner are the types of communicator a doctor must be at all times. Recognizing this, I have made a concerted effort to extend and to nurture my capacity for expressing my thoughts, making others experience them, and hearing out the thoughts and ideas of others.

Essay #9

"John, put another log on the fire." Sparks flew into the night sky. Only the front of me was warm. It was always like that, your back was always cold.

"You still want to be a doctor?"

I nodded.

"In this country you have to be the best. It's the hardest anywhere."

"Then I'll be the best."

"You must rely on yourself. I help as much as is possible, but here only the top get scholarship. In Poland it's easier, but here only a few get the whole shot. I think you can do it if you work hard."

"You know how I work when I want something."

"Yes, I know. Just take a day at a time and you'll do ok."

My father sipped his beer. Silence fell as we watched the flames dance on the logs.

As a young boy I would always look forward to camping with my father. Talk would fly over hundreds of topics as we walked through the forest or sat around the fire at night. He would ramble on about everything from his high blood pressure to nuclear reactions in the sun. Most of the time I never really understood all of what he said, yet I became charmed by the ideas, and thrilled when he would tell me something new. I wanted to know everything, but the more that I knew, the more I realized that I didn't know. Occasionally, I found this to be true too late, as unintentional explosions from my lab in the garage resulted in severe reprimands from my parents.

With age came moderation and a more formal road to education. The innocence of childhood tinkering had matured into the seriousness of adult tinkering, and with it the expectations I had of myself. Although my meager laboratory of childhood was no more, my love for the unknown was alive and well. In the real world though, things seldom went as smoothly as they had in the past.

"I can't get this experiment to work!" I would assert to myself while sitting at my lab bench. "Two o'clock in the morning and two weeks gone by. I swear I'll see these petri-dishes in my sleep. Dr. Youderian always said, 'This is what it's all about.' Indeed, perhaps this time. . ."

Those experiences when things didn't work were just as invaluable as those experiences when things did. After getting to know and appreciate the work and dedication required to discern even the smallest amount of information, it became clear to me why learning in the health sciences is truly lifelong.

Then there were those things which I found one learned only by doing. As a volunteer, I remember one night a young man my age came in with a knife wound to the chest.

"The lung is collapsed," the physician said. There was no time to anesthetize. Five people and myself held the patient down. As the physician made the incision, the boy writhed in pain. The screams made the hair on your neck stand up. As the blood spilled out onto the floor, you could see others around grimace and turn away.

"Look at that guy," I said to my friend nearby in a motion that indicated I was talking about the doctor. "Cool as a cucumber. Just another night at California Hospital for him."

I realized then that there was a lot more to medicine than getting an "A" in a class. I also realized that I still had a long way to go.

For now, that journey is really only beginning. I've taken "a day at a time," and as my father said years ago, I've done "ok." I've worked and planned for a long time, and it's gratifying, as well as slightly frightening, to see it all culminating so quickly now. During those years I hope I've grown and learned such that I might begin a career in medicine. I don't think I ever have been, or ever will be, the "best," but I do know that I've never stopped trying.

Essay #10

$\mathbf{M}$y career goal incorporates biomedical research, treating patients, and teaching. One person who has had particular influence upon this decision is Dr. Michelle Ehrlich. She is a pediatric neurologist who does extensive laboratory research in addition to treating patients. She is extremely effective in both parts of her career, and yet maintains activities outside her profession. Her ability to be a caring physician as well as a successful scientist has reinforced my desire to enter an M.D./Ph.D. program, where I feel I can best acquire the skills necessary for academic medicine.

Scientific research has always intrigued me, as have activities analogous to research, such as games and puzzles that require piecing together acquired items or facts. I enjoy reading the publications of the scientists I have been working with, observing how their results and conclusions evolve, and discussing where their research is heading. I experienced some of this often unpredictable research process myself last semester, while working in the Pharmacology department of the Cornell Veterinary College. In order to learn the techniques used in the lab, I investigated the effects of cobalt and cadmium ions on various properties of mast cells. Although the expected results were reasonably foreseeable, the actual results were not. What began as a laboratory exercise has ended up the topic of my senior honors thesis.

My enthusiasm for research extends beyond strictly basic science into the medical field. I have been working in basic science laboratories in clinical settings, both medical and veterinary. These experiences have stimulated my interest in the clinical applications of basic science research. As an academic physician, I would like to take my own research this one extra step, and have an influence upon the applications of my work. This would further enable me to interact with the patients I would be helping. Additionally, having been hospitalized several times myself, I know the value of a compassionate physician who will spend the extra few minutes explaining the patient's condition and what he or she can expect. Physicians and their patients often have very different ideas of what proper medical care entails, due to different values and beliefs, and it is vital that these differences be considered before any treatment is administered. Frequent patient communication would also help direct my research efforts by allowing me to detect any particular inadequacies in a given treatment and concentrate my work accordingly.

This type of interaction is important in teaching as well. As a teaching assistant for an introductory biology course, I enjoyed explaining ideas that fascinate me and found it particulary gratifying when a struggling student understood a concept with my help. I also liked challenging the more knowledgeable students during quizzes and discussions. They often came up with alternative explanations I had not thought of, teaching me as much as I taught them.

Eventually, I hope to practice medicine in an academic setting, in a position that combines research, teaching, and clinical practice. I feel that the combination of medical and graduate training offered by an M.D./Ph.D. program will enable me to attain this goal.

Essay #11

I spent my junior year of college at Queens' College, Cambridge University in England. There I studied chemistry and biochemistry (i.e. natural sciences). Credit for my coursework in England is to be applied toward my Cornell University B.A. degree. As of July 14, 1987, the final credit that I will receive for this work does not appear on my official transcript. Also, since I was abroad, I was not able to discuss with my faculty advisor which courses I should take during my senior year. Therefore, my academic record in this application is incomplete. I will notify AMCAS of corrections as soon as possible.

Summer activities:

1985—Volunteer at Pascack Valley Hospital Department of Radiology (Westwood, NJ). Helped with patients, aided x-ray and computer tomography technicians, ran errands for department supervisors.

1986—Lab technician at Rockefeller University (New York City). Conducted synthesis and purification of a protein tumor growth factor (co-researcher of paper pending publication).

1987—Continued research at Rockefeller University. Synthesized and examined analogs of tumor growth factor to discern relationship between structure and activity.

Essay #12

While exploring a wide range of activities, I discovered an increasing interest in the medical profession. Although desiring a general background, I felt drawn to this field by the challenge and opportunity to employ a variety of my skills and interests in benefitting others in an area of critical need. My love of animals and desire to help the rural worker originally drew me to veterinary medicine and the animal science major. However, after a year of college and exposure to rural areas lacking proper health care, I realized that a greater need existed for physicians.

Exposed to medicine early in life through my mother, a lab technician, and a brother, a doctor, I developed a natural curiosity that led from visits to my mother's lab to volunteering and later working in Clinical Pathology at Upstate. I rotated through the labs performing routine lab tests and became one of the few workers proficient in troubleshooting the equipment. To increase my contact with patients, I requested work as a morning blood-drawer and volunteered in the E.R. The time spent listening to and comforting the patients, especially the elderly, was invaluable.

At college, after performing RIA's for a year in an endocrinology research lab, I resolved to develop a safer assay. The next year was spent researching the alternate methods and finding professors interested in supporting my project. The ELISA method for progesterone in dogs I developed as an undergraduate research project then expanded into my honor's thesis.

Wanting to develop my other interests as well as pursue my goal to become a rural physician, I chose to continue with animal science, a flexible program offering many of the medically oriented courses. I developed a program strong in genetics and statistics while taking electives in the humanities and computers.

Through travel, reading, work, and various organizations, I pursued my other interests. My work as a computer teaching assistant and terminal operator this year will supplement my programming minor. To act on issues important to me, I joined AgPac, the Curriculum committee, and the campaign committees. Interested in international affairs, I was fortunate to be an Orientation Counselor to the entire International Living Center for foreign students. Enjoying the role of an O.C., I became a student advisor to 12 students, a position with similar but more lasting and personal responsibilities. To further improve my teaching skills, I offerred my services as a tutor through Ho-Nun-De-Kah and worked as a genetics teaching assistant responsible for a 30 student lab section. Riding since high school, I competed throughout the Northeast on the Cornell Riding Team and qualified for Regionals. My continuing interest in horses expanded into organizing horse shows, organizing public service symposiums, and teaching the handicapped to ride. My painting, drawing, and violin playing found an outlet through the various club activities.

These interests remained secondary to and contributed to a growing interest in the social problems facing rural areas. A summer working and living with a farm family and the many conversations we had concerning the difficulties of rural life, confirmed my desire to assist the rural community. At present I work for the Fresh Air Fund Camp which introduces intercity NYC poor and handicapped children to a healthy rural atmosphere while promoting respect for the farmer's role.

Farmers work 80 hour weeks in a high risk job without the benefit of retirement plans, medical plans, paid vacations, or paid sick days. Due to a low population density and thus political invisibility, rural areas frequently suffer from inadequate health care as they are unable to receive even the government support the urban poor receive. In addition, the long hours, understaffing, lack of modern facilities, and isolation in rural practices discourage many physicians.

Aware of these difficulties, I am committed to operating a clinic as a family practitioner, utilizing an effective support staff similar in organization to the Frontier Nursing Service. This practice allows the physicians to use their time more effectively in giving quality and humanistic care. It is my hope to establish such a clinic in a rural area presently lacking in health care.

Essay #13

Adversity was my transition to maturity. Freshman year was marked by an academic citation, election to dorm council and close friends, but it was also a time of misfortune. I was suspended for three weeks for disorderly conduct due to excessive drinking. As a former dorm proctor, church altar boy and Eagle Scout, I had virtually no experience with drinking. When I returned, I trained as an Alcohol Peer Counselor, and later realized that Dartmouth's party atmosphere was inappropriate for me.

I applied to Northwestern and Cornell. Northwestern immediately accepted me; Cornell accepted me for January admission. After a successful term at Northwestern, I was pleased to join my brother at Cornell and receive a generous scholarship. In addition, Cornell selected me a Transfer Fellow due to my academic and extracurricular record.

Some students with a distruped start as a freshman might give up any aspiration of becoming a doctor. The goal, however, was too important to me. I first considered becoming a doctor ten years ago. I participated in a gifted program at a nearby university. In a biology course, we dissected various organs, wore surgical gloves, and worked with scalpels. I loved it.

During this same time my grandfather, who lived with us, was told he had terminal cancer. He changed from a strong, healthy man to an emaciated skeleton. I recall the helplessness I felt as I watched him slowly die. At twelve, I decided to become a physician.

I examined my ambition more seriously in high school. I founded the Hotchkiss Medical Club. We met many doctors and went on trips to Bridgeport Hospital and Yale University. Everything about medicine fascinated me.

At seventeen I confronted a medical emergency. Mother and I were driving into a shopping center. The driver in the car ahead suddenly slumped over the wheel. I pulled the old, bearded man out of the car and administered CPR. When the ambulance crew arrived, I continued while they did other things to revive the patient. Since then, as a lifeguard at a busy state park, I saved lives; and, as a Red Cross volunteer, I assisted in emergency rooms.

As a senior, I look back on my freshman experience with a

new understanding. People make mistakes. What you do with your life after a setback shows your true worth. As an Alcohol Peer Counselor, I educated others about the perils of excessive drinking. At Northwestern and Cornell, I helped establish similar programs. As a Residential Advisor, Peer Educator, and counselor, I helped freshmen avoid dumb mistakes. In turn, I learned to assist peers with problems of depression, rape, drug abuse, unwanted pregnancy and homosexuality. As an Administrative Orientation Counselor, I trained counselors in listening, leadership, and human relations. Recently, I was selected to the University Hearing Board because of my record of leadership, ethical standards, and genuine concern for others. All of my experiences, both positive and negative, prepared me for the maturity, responsibility, and sensitivity demanded of a physician.

Essay #14

To work with people, to help them when they are sick, and to find ways to prevent illnesses is a challenge. When I volunteered at the Virginia Home for the Disabled in Richmond, I often felt that many illnesses were preventable. I also had the opportunity to help my father treat patients, and I was always thrilled by the successful administration of medicine.

Academic preparation for medical school initially dominated my school career at the University of Richmond. However, in the last year I, under the tutelage of a professor at the University of Richmond, found myself very involved in a research program which resulted in the publication of a paper. This program taught me how to maintain endurance and interest in an academic area and was therefore the most educational experience in my college career. My communicative and persuasive skills were also developed, for the research involved the competitive procurement of grants as well as the lecturing to audiences of varying backgrounds on the subject matter.

As a result of the emphasis on the research project, I did not take all of the courses required for premedical preparation, but I had an unexpected opportunity to compensate the following year. My original plan was to join the Peace Corps between college and medical school. I succeeded in graduating (cum laude) early. Unfortunately the assignment was delayed for more than a year. It was during this time that I continued to carry on my interest in research. I worked as a laboratory technician and as an assistant in an OB-GYN practice. As a technician in a private laboratory in Massachusetts, I was able to perform supervised experiments in order to identify and isolate clotting factors in Horseshoe crab blood—with possible implications of medicinal value.

Upon moving to Virginia, I began a part-time occupation in an OB-GYN practice. Working in a medical practice has made me realize that the need for communicating information is just as vital as learning it. Therefore, I have tried to prepare myself in this area as well. Being raised in a bilingual (American/German) household, I am at ease in speaking either language. I added Spanish during my first year in college at St. Louis University in Madrid, Spain. Further, being somewhat of a history buff has allowed me to extend my communicative skills as well:

I am currently an active docent for the Fairfax County Park Authority, and thus I give tours at a representative Virginia plantation named Sully.

To some extent travel allowed me insight into the culture, religion, and needs of other people. In addition, another very enlightening experience occurred during the summer of 1983 in Woods Hole, Massachusetts. I partook in a marine research program given by Boston University and was confronted with a vast new area of information in both historic and scientific respects. The summer courses centered on detailed studies and independent research projects dealing with the oceans and their inhabitants. Emphasis was also placed on the individual's ability to cooperate and to withstand the physical hardships that a small crowded sailing vessel foisted upon one. My research project on this cruise resulted in a paper on the polychaete population in the Bay of Fundy.

My recreational hobbies include a wide variety of non-medically oriented activities. For example, I am learning how to play the classical guitar. I maintain a productive herb and flower graden. I enjoy windsurfing in the local waters. During the winter months, I also spend a great deal of time involved in ice skating, skiing, wood carving, and needlecraft. Furthermore, I sew most of my wardrobe. I have been involved with jewelry making, with mechanical car repairs, and with the German School Choir. I also learned some veterinary medicine when my entire family took a summer course at Cornell University Adult Education.

My life has been exciting and diversified. Evenso, I have never lost sight of the quest to become a physician.

Essay #15

My interest in medicine is rooted in various medically related positions I have held in clinical and research settings. In 1982 I was awarded an NIH summer fellowship at Roswell Park Memorial Institute, Buffalo, New York, where I characterized an anti leukemia-lymphoma monoclonal antibody. This work won the institute's Sydney Farber Award for Outstanding Independent Research. Conducting research in a laboratory associated with several hospitals offered insights into the relationship between basic science and health care. The following summer I worked as a dissector for the Department of Anatomy, State University of New York at Buffalo Medical School, preparing prosections for the gross anatomy course. I enjoyed both the analytical approach of laboratory research and the precision of dissection: hence I sought further experience in the biomedical field.

During my freshman year at Cornell I applied to the College Scholar Program as a means of combining interests in the biological and social sciences. Under the auspices of this program, competitively selected undergraduates design their own majors, integrating broad topics not accommodated by the usual curriculum. I am pursuing concentrations in cell biology and Soviet studies.

In the summer of 1984 I worked as an emergency room volunteer at the Buffalo General Hospital. At the same time, as a Summer Research Fellow at the Department of Oral Biology, State University of New York at Buffalo Dental School, I prepared monoclonal antibodies against the oral pathogen *Actinobacillus actinomycetemcomitans*. These antibodies have since been patented by the university. This intensive, simultaneous exposure to biomedical reseach and clinical practice firmly established my resolve to pursue a career in medicine. It also persuaded me of the importance of research as a foundation underlying medical practice; consequently I have used the flexibility of the College Scholar Program to integrate research into my academic work. I substituted an independent research project of characterizing an *Apium graviolens* enzyme, in the course of which I used most basic biochemical techniques, for the traditional biochemistry lab course. Upon completion of this project I began research on the structure and function of glucose-6-phosphatase in conjunction with work being performed in the laboratory of Dr. William Arion, Department of Biochemistry, Molecular and Cell Biology, Cornell University.

Currently I am participating in the DeBakey Summer Program at the Department of Surgery, Baylor College of Medicine. I assist in cardiovascular surgery under Dr. E. Stanley Crawford at the Methodist Hospital of Houston, and work during my free time at the emergency room and trauma center of the nearby Benjamin Taub county hospital. Through this experience I have learned, by direct participation, aspects of the day-to-day reality of cardiovascular surgery and trauma care; happily found myself capable of maintaining a first year intern's hours; and, by working with patients in two so vastly different institutions, have been stimulated to reconsider some social aspects of the health care delivery system.

Essay #16

My interest in becoming a physician has developed through exposure to both clinical medicine and investigative research. In the first area, I have had the opportunity to work in the office practice of an ophthalmologist and to observe surgery at three hospitals. In college, I successfully completed an Emergency Medical Technician training course. Throughout these experiences, I was impressed and inspired by the skill, dedication and compassion of the professionals with whom I worked and studied.

I was introduced to investigative medicine during an eight-week paid fellowship in the Tissue Typing Laboratory of the New York Blood Center. In this position I learned the basic histocompatability tests necessary to match donors with recipients for kidney and bone marrow transplantation and studied the relationship between specific HLA factors and certain diseases such as Juvenile Macular Degeneration.

With a strong recommendation from the Blood Center, I procured a salaried position of greater scientific complexity and responsibility at Memorial Cancer Center in the Summer of 1984. My extensive work in the immunohematology laboratory of Memorial has been the single most significant force in my decision to attend medical school.

The first summer I was responsible for establishment and maintainance of several of the first cell lines derived from patients with Acquired Immunodeficiency Syndrome (AIDS) and the analysis of AIDS patients' immune response through measurement of lymphocyte transformation and Natural Killer Cell activity *in vitro*. I was the only student approved to work in the P-3, biological containment level, laboratory that year.

In 1984, there was very little documentation concerning the transmission and prognosis of AIDS. Our research was directed at determining the efficacy of several drugs in restoring AIDS patients' immune response. Although I was working with patient blood in a high-containment facility and had realistic concerns for the safety of myself and others working in the laboratory, I felt extremely fortunate to have the opportunity to use my recently acquired skills and to learn new procedures within a formal research design. My greatest satisfaction was observing the connection between what we were accomplishing in the laboratory and the plight of the AIDS patients with whom I met and talked.

During the following January, I returned to the immunohematology laboratory at Memorial where I was given the opportunity to continue with my work at a more sophisticated level and with more independence. My research during this month was aimed at determining whether the antigenic agent recognized when normal Natural Killer cells lyse AIDS target cells is similar to the antigen expressed by Epstein-Barr virus-infected cells.

This past summer I returned again to the laboratory to assist in supervising and was assigned to train new members of the team, one of whom was a doctor doing a fellowship in our laboratory. This was the summer of the greatest recognition of the importance of the AIDS virus and anxiety about transmission into the population outside the previously accepted high-risk groups. Strengthening the containment levels and adding additional precautions, I tested a newly proposed drug for AIDS, investigated the cell-mediated immunity of growth hormone-deficient patients, continued to maintain cell lines and learned a new interferon assay.

While I plan to defer my decision as to which field I will specialize in until after completion of my basic science studies, my experience at Memorial over the last two years has convinced me of my aptitude and interest in investigative research. However, in whatever field I choose, I will not divorce myself from patient care, for it was the personal interaction with patients that made my laboratory experience most meaningful.

Essay #17

My interests in biomedical science and the performing arts developed while I was a youngster. Fortunately, I have been able to enjoy both fields.

Since May 1985, I have been working part-time during classes and full-time during breaks as a research technician at NIH, in Dr. John E. Folk's group (Natl. Inst. of Dental Research, Laboratory of Oral Biology and Physiology, Enzyme Chemistry Section). I assist Dr. Myung Hee Park. The focus of our work is one of the eukaryotic protein synthesis initiation factors, eIf-4D, a protein which contains the unusual amino acid hypusine (N -(4-amino-2-hydroxybutyl)lysine) as the result of post-translational modification: a lysine residue receives the butylamine portion of spermidine and is subsequently hydroxylated. The functions of the factor and its hypusine residue are unknown at this time. In Sept. 1985, I was assigned my own project, the molecular cloning and sequencing of cDNA coding for eIF-4D. A bacteriophage lambda gt11 human hepatoma expression library was screened with oligonucleotide and antibody probes, and DNA sequencing experiments are currently underway. During the summer of 1985, I was engaged in the purification of eIF-4D from human erythrocytes by multistep chromatography and differential precipitation, analyzing the product by SDS-PAGE, LPLC and amino acid analysis. I am a coauthor of two papers and one abstract which describe that summer's work.

At George Mason University, I worked from Dec. 1983 to Sept. 1984 as research assistant to Prof. Suzanne Slayden of the Chemistry Department, studying the competition between protonolysis and rearrangement in certain trialkylboranes. In addition to learning the required air-sensitive techniques, I routinely analyzed the products using GC and proton NMR. From Aug. 1984 to the present, I have been working with Dr. Slayden on a series of instructional videotapes designed to introduce various forms of spectroscopy to students of organic chemistry. These programs feature computer graphics and animations which I created in my spare time. One of them—"Interpreting NMR Spectra"—will be presented at the American Chemical Society's Mid-Atlantic Regional Meeting in Baltimore.

Prior to my return to college, I worked from Jan. 1980 to July

1983 as a Senior Research Technician at The New York Blood
Center, assisting Dr. Bernard Horowitz of the Blood Deriva-
tives Program. Dr. Horowitz provided me with a working tutor-
ial in experimental and process-scale protein chemistry, and
eventually encouraged me to complete my formal education.
My first year in his lab produced a chromatographic method
for the purification of human leukocyte interferons. I characterized the material using isoelectric focusing, SDS-PAGE and
2D-PAGE, comparing the distribution of interferon subtypes in
the highly-purified chromatographic eluate to those in the non-
recombinant interferon preparations then approved for use in
human clinical trials. My efforts were then directed to the purification and characterization of human Factor VIII:C. Its association with von Willebrand factor was probed, and a number
of RIAs and ELISAs were developed. The final phase of my
work with Dr. Horowitz grew out of the AIDS epidemic: I investigated several methods of chemically inactivating viruses
in blood products, aiming for conditions which were benign to
Factor VIII procoagulant activity, yet left the injectables
virus- and reagent-free. This project was passed on to other
workers when I returned to school. I was a coauthor of two abstracts describing some of the interferon and Factor VIII work.

My laboratory experience also includes eighteen months
(1978-80) as a clinical laboratory technician at Pathology
Associates Laboratories in Beverly Hills, CA. I was responsible
for running the daily "panel" of blood chemistries on an auto-
mated analyzer and flame photometer, and routinely performed
RIAs and inoculated cultures. Other ongoing duties included
the preparation of samples and the logging of patient information. I was intially hired as a courier by this lab, but was pro-
moted into the laboratory at my request.

From 1971 to 1978, I was a performer (actor, singer and
guitarist). I appeared in three Broadway shows, four national
tours and numerous radio and television broadcasts. My association with the pathology lab started as one of the many jobs
between shows, but proved to be the beginning of a new and
more satisfying career, one free of the cyclic unemployment of
the actor's life. My training in drama and music has proven to
be a valuable asset in the biomedical field: an actor is taught
to prepare and empathize; a musician develops manual dexterity and structured study habits; both must adapt to a wide
variety of environments, and both require the ability to work in
tandem with people of diverse backgrounds and interests.

Essay #18

I have wanted to become a doctor since I first watched my ophthalmologist father treat patients and since I learned that I was born with a tracheo-esophogeal fistula, and first wondered at the miracle of modern medicine that had occurred inside my own body. Yet, these realities have very little to do with my desire to become a physician today: over the past several years, an intuition has been transformed into an informed, intellectual motivation.

I spent two summers during high school as a volunteer counselor at ANCHOR, a camp for emotionally, physically, and mentally handicapped children and adults in New York. The work was demanding (I spent hours each day lifting arms and legs during exercise classes, helping women change into swim-suits for the beach, running after missing campers) and emo-tionally challenging (many of the men and women were verbal-ly abusive and physically threatening—more of them were depressed) but, by the end of my first summer, a camper whom I had been guiding had gained enough confidence to step into the pool on a hot day: this was all the reward I needed.

Eager to explore the psychological and psychiatric problems that I have encountered recreationally, in the summer after my Freshman year, I worked at Payne Whitney Hospital as a research assistant on an NIMH study of the effectiveness of family therapy intervention for inpatients with schizophrenia and major affective disorders. I tabulated data, contacted sub-jects, performed follow-up interviews, observed group therapy, attended team conferences and made rounds with the residents and senior staff. I experienced some of the challenges of research: I saw instances where the protocol came into conflict with a patient's best interest; I realized how challenging it could be to get subjects to maintain their commitment to the project. I observed many of the frustrations and rewards of clinical psychiatry: in the last week of the summer one patient tried to commit suicide for the fourth time and another went home to her family and her job.

The following summer, I worked on a NIH study of juvenile macular degeneration at Manhattan Eye, Ear, Nose and Throat Hospital. I had designed a statistical form for diagnosis re-trieval and was assisting in the epidemiological study when the staff nurses and ancillary personnel at the hospital walked out on a strike. Since I had recently completed an emergency medical technician training course, I volunteered to substitute for striking workers in the emergency department. The emergency room held wonders that I had not imagined from the seclusion of the retinal research laboratory upstairs: I tested the visual acuity of elderly women with glaucoma and of people who spoke only Spanish or Polish or Greek; I listened to the fears of a concerned parent of an infant with a corneal ulcer; I comforted a young girl who was having a cockroach removed from her ear; I explained the importance of self-assessment vision testing to a man with macular degeneration. When a woman walked in one night with an orbital fracture and a facial laceration, I held her hand as the plastic surgeon placed fifteen stitches in her cheek. I stopped a woman as she tried to snap a leather belt in front of the eyes of her pre-school child: the resident had just treated him for a corneal abrasion. Through the otoscope and the slit-lamp biomicroscope—on my first day—I saw a ruptured ear drum and a herpes dendritic corneal ulcer. From week to week as patients returned for follow-up examinations, I tested their visual acuity and excitedly watched the return of their vision.

Also at MEETH, I witnessed the struggles of people who could not afford to purchase medical care. I spoke with a man who had allowed his pterygium to progress beyond the point of reversible sight loss: he told me that he had waited to come in because he knew he would not be able to pay. Throughout the summer, many of the complexities of health care provision for a diverse group of patients became evident to me: I lost an image of my father treating macula patients in his office and gained a more complicated and, for me, more fascinating portrait of medical care. To assimilate my new ideas, I enrolled at the London School of Economics for a year's study of social policy and health administration.

In London and at the LSE, I studied and searched for answers to some of the questions I had posed while working in the emergency room. At Williams I had trained to be a contraception and health counselor to my peers: at the LES, I studied family planning policies in the United States, the United Kingdom, and China. As I sat in the offices of my health care administration professors—all of whom had advisory positions within the National Health Service—I rediscovered a personal talent that had been overshadowed by years of English and pre-medical courses. At Horace Mann High School, I had distinguished myself in organization and leadership as the elected Chairman of both the Allocations Committee and the Governing Council. At Williams, I had been selected by the college president to serve as one of three student representatives on the board of Trustees' Committee on Priorities and Resources. At the LSE, I learned that what had enabled me to work effectively on these committees was essential to the role of health policy, breastfeeding in the Third World, provision of emergency care in the NHS and the relationship between race and health and I wrote papers and delivered class lectures with an interest that was unparalleled in all of my past academic work.

Yet, for all the gratification and intellectual excitement I found studying health care administration, I never discarded my intention to become a doctor: rather, my experience has more firmly convinced me of the correctness of my choice. Now, I am prepared and anxious to study medicine with a full awareness that medical decisions and problems have social and political roots and implications and a full consciousness of the essential humanity of medical practice.

Essay #19

I have never understood the great hullabaloo some people raise about a conflict between science and the humanities. All my life I have been attracted to both and am puzzled by the perspective of a friend who claims, "I'm not a 'science person,'" or some of my fraternity brothers who raise their brows when I register for a class in poetry writing. As a profession, I feel medicine will allow me to live in both worlds.

I enjoy learning about lots of different things, so school has always been easy and fun. I also take great pride in being competent in many areas, from basketball and windsurfing to tutoring math and cooking chicken paprikash. For as long as I can remember, I have been an addict of the animal shows appearing on television. I love watching polar bears plunging through ice and close-ups of frogs laying jelly-covered eggs. But I never aspired to be shooting those films, knee deep in mire or perched in a tree, and I don't want to be a veterinarian. When I first entered high school I wanted to direct films, modeling myself after Francois Truffaut. Later I decided I would satisfy this desire with artful home movies or perhaps by assisting in a medical documentary. Writing fiction is one of my favorite hobbies and I would love, some day, to try publishing a novel.

Of all my interests, I have a special passion for biology which I expect everyone to share. The magic in living things which transcends molecular and cellular analysis makes studying them the most interesting thing I can imagine. So when someone blurts, "Ugh! I hated biology in high school!" I smile but honestly wonder if he is crazy. My research experience of two summers in a neuroimmunology lab at Columbia intensified this conviction and made me even more excited about my plans to study medicine.

There is a tradition of doctors on both the Cuban and Hungarian sides of my family, but it was only late in high school that I decided for sure that I wanted to study medicine myself. When my older brtother, now studying at Mount Sinai, decided to go into medicine, I chose all my high school courses in areas outside natural science. Gradually, I realized that I could still like science, or consider a medical career, without just copying my brother. Volunteering in the emergency room at Columbia Presbyterian last summer was the final step I needed to evaluate my commitment to medicine and it has made me sure that I am doing the right thing. I sought out the smelliest and bloodiest patients, changing their bed pans and bringing them water, and once helped restrain a woman having heart seizures while blood streamed from a catheter in her nose. I found that actively helping made these experiences less and less gross and unexpectedly emboldened me to tackle something bigger. I was also inspired by the exciting side of medicine, rushing to the trauma room in any free moment to watch the surgeons clean and stitch wounds. Sometimes I caught myself grinning on the subway ride home, wondering if some day I would be sewing wounds myself.

Though I welcome excitement and intellectual satisfaction, what I really want from my career is to feel I am channeling a lifetime of energy into something meaningful and worthwhile. As compared to a career in business, or directing films, I believe studying and practicing medicine will fulfill this need. The greatest asset I have to offer is my motivation, to give and to work, to become as good a doctor as I am able to. Beside a warm family and close friends, there is truly nothing I want more and nothing that would make me happier.

Essay #20

bad

The rate at which medical knowledge is moving along today has brought out the necessity for two very important qualities in physicians: an open mind, which will recognize the advantages and, at the same time, limitations of new technologies and practising methods, and a high degree of adaptability, which will allow these new methods to be effectively integrated into medical practice.

I believe that my life experience reflects such qualities. Throughout my education I have tried to keep an open mind and expand my horizons. Making the decision to come to the United States for my college education was a step in that direction. Prior to that, I had spent significant periods of time in Africa (Zambia, Ghana and Morocco), and in travelling through Europe. My stay in Morocco was particularly interesting: I witnessed the efforts of an ambitious ruler to inspire a fascinating but at times distorting process of modernization along western models.

I spent the latter part of my schooling at Campion School in Athens, Greece, which prepares students according to the British educational system. Although my high school community was small and rather close-knit, its environment was limiting only to those who chose to find limits in themselves. Besides my placing first in my graduating class, I was active in student government, classical drama, three varsity sports, and classical guitar performances. At the same time I came to develop a keen interest in the biological sciences and a fascination for the humanitarian aspects of medicine.

Coming to the University of Pennsylvania to explore the field of Biology was a major decision which I took conscious of the new directions it would open up for me. The environment was quite different from any other I had known before, but I needed the challenge to see how valuable my previous experiences really were. After all, my intention had always been to build for myself a perspective which would give me a good degree of awareness and adaptability. Admission to the highly competitive University Scholars program and my success in gaining a place on the varsity soccer team placed me in a very challenging milieu within the university. I believe I responded well. Academically, my program of liberal arts studies reached deep into the process of intellectual enrichment which I consider to be basic to the notion of scholarship. In sports, I became the top varsity goal scorer in the 1984-1985 season and was voted most improved player.

My motivation is a tool which I love to put to use in causes that I feel are worthwhile. This is reflected in the significant broadening of activities at the Penn Greek Club since December, 1985, when I took office as President. We began to organize a series of lectures and films on issues as diverse as recent political developments in Greece, the restoration of Athenian monuments, and the Olympic theme. The response was quite rewarding: our club membership eventually tripled.

I have come to regard medicine as a field where the practitioner is in a constant, intimate relationship with science while drawing on much more than just pure science. This dialectic process holds a special appeal for me. In my mind, emphasis in medical care should be as much on "care" as on the "medical" or scientific aspect. Furthermore, I recognize medicine as a field flexible enough for one to follow his own particular course, and even open up new ways. I see, for example, that in the future the dedicated physician may need to become more and more associated to the statesman and the law-maker; the effects that medical advances have in shaping society and culture are too great for medicine to be regarded solely as an intellectual enterprise. This of course entails expanded responsibilities. I feel capable of contributing to the undertaking.

Essay #21

During the past year, as I was finalizing decisions about my career choice I have had to accept a more realistic picture of the medical profession than one I had in the past. Based on talks I have had with some physicians, I have gained a better understanding of some of the current problems in medicine. I have also gained a better appreciation of the dedication and devotion of these physicians. These conversations, which at first shocked me, eventually fueled a growing interest that I had in medicine.

Though a medical career had been a consideration since high school, it remained one of several considerations until I began to concentrate in the sciences and accumulate some experience in the area during college.

During the summer of my sophomore year at Cornell, I worked in a reagents research and development lab for a supplier of hospital diagnostic equipment. After deriving improved reagents for spectrophotometric blood analyzers, I tested the accuracy of the new formulas. My summer at Instrumentation Labs proved helpful in future work because I had a chance to familiarize myself with a more sophisticated lab.

In the spring of my junior year I worked with Dr. W.R. Butler of the Physiology Department at Cornell, researching endogenous opiates in rats. In addition to localizing a source of the opiates in the adrenal medulla, I was able to achieve an acetylcholine dependant surge in opiate secretion from the adrenal. Dr. Butler guided me in establishing a credible experimental design, and technicians have introduced me to a number of relevant assay techniques. In the fall, I will be investigating the possible role of opiates integrated with pituitary and/or hypothalamic hormones in regulating the stress response of rats.

This past summer I worked in the Thyroid Diagnostic Center of the Brigham and Women's Hospital for Dr. P.R. Larsen, director of the unit, and Dr. Ira Mills, a Ph.D. doing postdoctoral work in endocrinology. I studied deiodination of thyroid hormone (mainly in the form of T4) to triiodothyronine (T3). T3 has been shown to be a much more active form of the hormone, but T4 is the more predominant thyroid product, thus the conversion is important physiologically. An enzyme similar to the one responsible for the deiodination leading to most of the circulating T3 has been found in brown adipose tissue and may be involved in non-shivering thermogenesis. I investigated the effects of various hormonal treatments on this enzymatically mediated conversion and described receptor mechanisms operating in isolated cells. I have learned conventional biochemical lab procedures, such as RIA's and electrophoresis techniques, and have also had the chance to absorb some of the expertise of the physicians and Ph.D's with whom I have worked. Additionally, while at Brigham and Women's, I have attended lectures given by hospital and lab personnel.

This recent experience has served to focus my career interests. While in school I have enjoyed studying endocrinology and immunology, and I would like to go on to study internal medicine. Eventually, I want to work in a university affiliated hospital, and to be involved in clinically related research, while maintaining patient contact.

At Cornell I have probed some of my other interests, including economics, psychology and politics, as well as taken rigorous science courses which have prepared me well for the demanding curriculum at medical school. I have been an ambassador for the Arts and Sciences School for the past two years during which I have housed prospective Cornellians and have given tours to their families. Also, as a Biology Student Advisor, I have been responsible for advising a group of ten freshmen each year about the biology program at Cornell. In the 1986-87 school year I will be a Resident Advisor in a predominantly freshman dorm. I expect the challenges and rewards to be tremendous.

Medicine interests me because it is often adjusting to new technology and ideas. A career in medicine excites me, not only because of my interests but because it is an opportunity for me to do something I think I could do well while deriving the gratification that comes from helping people.

Essay #22

I find myself trying to answer the question "Why do you want to be a doctor?" Such a question seems to demand an organized and logical response which I can produce without much trouble, but which is only answers instead of reasons: "I am interested in sciences; I like people; I think it would be exciting." My own answer to myself is more simple, yet more inexplicable—simply that the closer I get to medical practice, the more I like it and the better "gut-feeling" I get about my decision to pursue it. It is our feelings we react to, the justification comes afterwards. Thus I find myself only able to offer a logical rationalization of the emotional responses that are my actual motivation to pursue medicine.

In contrast to many of my fellow pre-meds at Cornell, I entered college with no intention of ever pursuing medicine as a career. I had always been interested in wildlife and environmental studies. I travelled as far as Maine and Alaska in ecological study programs. I taught myself taxidermy and museum preservation skills. In fact it was Cornell's reputation in ornithology that led me to Ithaca. Yet as I became more deeply involved in animal behavior studies, I started to feel a nagging uncertainty as to whether wildlife research was indeed all that I wanted. Realizing that I might be continuing in this study more by inertia than conviction, I decided to take a semester leave of absence to assist a Cornell doctoral student in his research on mockingbird behavior in Texas, hoping to decide whether I really wanted to continue in this direction. After a month or two of this research, I found that the aesthetics of the environment still moved me, but everyday we were working on the same problem, and it quickly became apparent that the results could never justify the effort to me. I grew frustrated with the often myopic intensity of this form of research, and the way an individual's success or failure seemed to depend only on the substance of his thesis, to the apparent exclusion of the content of his character.

Having abandoned what I had always assumed would be my destined career, I used much of my free time in Texas for introspection and soulsearching, trying to decide what I wanted and valued in my life. It was a fascination with science that drew me into biology originally, and though pure research appears too tightly focused to satisfy me, I still enjoy studying science immensely. But I also know that science means more to me if it is linked to individual people. I have decided that medicine or teaching would be the best way for me to stay involved in science, since each incorporates the humanistic qualities that pure research has not seemed to require; and knowing myself, I think that I will be more happy as the doctor rather than the teacher.

My experience this summer has given me added confidence in my decision to pursue medicine. I have been working as a surgical scrub tech in the Johns Hopkins Hospital Gynecology Operating Room. Every day I am scrubbed and in the middle of surgery, sometimes for six hours at a time, handing instruments, threading sutures, retracting, and always asking questions. I have never enjoyed a job more and I truly can't think of anything I would rather be doing this summer, (and certainly nothing else that would get me out of bed at 5:30 a.m. every day). Even when I know nothing about the patient, the science and the surgical technique are fascinating, but when I can talk to the patient and develop at least some personal contact, the science suddenly becomes medicine and it takes on new meaning, for it is that personal contact that moves me the most.

When Helen Avery said good-bye to me for this summer with tears in her eyes, saying she didn't know what she was going to do without me, I realized the feeling that is probably my strongest motivation. She is 87 years old, with two artificial knees, and the beginnings of Parkinson's disease, but she is still the sharpest of all the elderly that I visited last year. Every Friday afternoon I went to see her, sometimes to go for a walk, sometimes to take her shopping, but mostly just to talk. I cannot describe how good it felt to know that my presence mattered, to see her light up and smile when she opened the door for me. As a doctor, hopefully, I can find that feeling again and again. The science may interest me, the diagnoses may challenge me, but it will be that personal involvement with the patient that will make the most difference to me and keep me going through the hardest parts.

My interest in the field of medicine is the product of a life-long process of discovery which began when I was a child. My mother, a clinical pathologist, and my father, a research pathologist, were responsible for many of the early experiences which sparked my interest in medicine. Through such experiences, I was exposed to many facets of the field, from wonderous triumphs to harsh realities. As a child, I would frequently visit my parents' laboratories. My father would demonstrate the uses of many modern pieces of equipment, often allowing me to look through his electron microscope, while my mother would show me her patients' slides, explaining the reasons for the various and too often malignant diagnoses.

My summer experiences have given me several opportunities to examine the field of medicine first-hand. During the past three summers, I have worked at NYU Medical Center on projects which have provided me with some perspective on both the clinical and basic-science aspects of medicine. At the Rusk Institute, I worked with a team which rehabilitated stroke and accident victims, both physically and emotionally, and I thus became familiar with some of the basic requirements of patient care. In the Department of Hematology, my research for the past two summers focused on the glycoprotein IIb-IIIa complex, which comprises the fibrinogen receptor site on the surface of the platelet membrane. One aspect of this research dealt with investigating the mechanism of Post Transfusion Purpura, a platelet incompatability disorder caused by PLA_1, an antigen present on most individuals' glycoprotein IIIa. Consequently, I performed numerous experiments utilizing electrophoresis techniques as well as monoclonal antibodies in Western Blot procedures.

While these projects have served to confirm the intellectual basis for my interest in medicine, non-academic events have shaped my emotional commitment to the field. Through my three-year participation in the Veterans Administration Hospital Volunteers Program, I have derived immense satisfaction by providing conversation and companionship to lonely elderly patients and younger veterans with psychiatric disorders. At the Rusk Institute, I was able to witness and share in the joy patients feel upon slowly regaining strength in their limbs. All of these experiences have made me dramatically aware that physicians have an unparalleled opportunity to help others; this prospect, more than any other, has become my major inducement towards a career as a physician.

Essay #24

I have been a springboard diver for half of my life. I started at age ten, and by the time I was thirteen I was training six days a week, not because my coach or my parents told me to, but because I loved it. Diving has been my most consistent undertaking over the years; it is the unifying thread that has not only given me immense pleasure, but that has also helped me to grow and to become the person I want to be. As I look back, I see the few material gains diving has given me, such as travel and college offers, but more importantly, I see the vast personal gains it has provided: The ability to do hard work, the ability to honor a committment, the mastery of fear, the experiences of success and self-confidence, and the ability to achieve, to be successful in the face of competition, the ability to sacrifice to achieve the goals I have set.

Diving has given me much, but it has not always been fun. The competition and the mastery of a new dive are what make the sport worthwhile for me, but to achieve these moments of beauty, long hours of practice are necessary—through the winter months, through the times when my friends were out enjoying themselves, through the times when I was not well or was tired. To succeed, I have had to set hard, specific goals for myself, such as becoming a High School All-American (which I achieved), winning the New York State Empire Games (which I did), qualifying for the NCAA Division I Championships (which I have not yet done), and becoming an NCAA All-American (which I most probably will never be). When I think about sleeping and missing a morning workout, or going off with my friends, I recall my goals and realize that I need every bit of practice I can get. Diving has made me realize something that guides me throughout my life: If I want to achieve badly enough, I must make sacrifices now to reach my goals.

As I have progressed, I have gained self-confidence and pride from my ability to work hard for what I want. Also, I have over and over conquered an emotion that feels good to conquer, fear; fear of hitting the board, fear of hitting the water, fear of being out of control 33 feet in the air, fear of performing and exposing my inner self to crowds, fear of failure. I, and all other divers, have experienced all these, many times over. I have really hurt myself, really embarassed myself. What has been most important to me, though, is the ability I have gained to force myself back up there, to try the dive again, to dive in front of the same old crowd the next week. When I can, and can later succeed, the fear goes away, and the confidence in overcoming the fear grows.

Diving has taught me, too, the concept of balance. In college we work out from three to five hours a day, and from December to March have long trips to compete elsewhere. I, like all athletes, have learned how to study when I am tired after workouts. I have learned how to dive and live my life at the same time, how to study and have fun while upholding the athletic standards I have chosen. I have also learned how to maintain my body and my mind, how to elicit the best performance possible, and how to remain healthy when my performance or the team's success depends on it. I have learned to think when I am tired.

I have been successful at the sport, and it has influenced my way of life and my ways of thinking. I believe the qualities that I have gained from diving will help me to be successful in medicine. I have the ability to work hard, experience physical discomfort and mental fatigue, and continue to think and perform well. I can make sacrifices to achieve goals I believe in. I believe that I have the maturity and emotional stability to cope with the rigors of a doctor's education and life, and the personal integrity that will enable me to uphold the trust and responsibility placed in a doctor. And I will always retain my sense of balance—to take all that life can throw at me and turn it to my best advantage. Diving and medicine are both paradoxical—one must strive for perfection, but must realize that perfection will never be reached. To succeed in medicine is my main goal for the rest of my life; it is a goal I believe I can achieve.

Essay #25

My growing up in a medical family was probably what provided the initial impetus for my interest in a medical career. However, it is my own experiences, apart from my family, which have made it clear to me that this choice is truly based on what I want to do with my life.

My mother is a physician and she has provided a meaningful role model for me. I was aware throughout, of her ability to combine concern for helping people with their medical problems with a strong concern for each individual. I was impressed with her investment in seeing that each patient received the best possible medical care and her ability to combine patient care with ongoing research—research which led to some significant contributions in the area of treatment. My father's position, as I was growing up, as the Medicaid administrator for the city, brought home to me the issues related to equitable delivery of medical care. His devotion of much of his adult life to a program that was a step in the direction of providing medical care for all people in need, regardless of income or insurance regulations, has hopefully made a difference in people's lives.

It is the experiences which I have had, however, which have been important in furthering my understanding of the complexities and realities of the life of a physician. The volunteer work which I did at the Health Sciences Center exposed me to the kind of research which needs to be ongoing in relation to medical problems, and which ultimately contributes to improved patient care. The painstaking work which I was engaged in, in translating CAT scan data onto computers was part of an attempt to clarify how bone conformation relates to locomotion. I can see such data being used in a variety of preventive ways—as for example, in rehabilitation after injuries, in determining the amount of stress an athlete can withstand and in cases of osteroperosis, among others.

My work in the Orthopedic Department at County Medical Center has shown me even more sharply than any previous experience, the complex nature of the skills which contribute to making the competent, caring physician. The in-depth understanding of the human body, the complicated skills needed in performing surgery and the need to find ways of dealing with the tragedies which physicians are confronted with, present a lifelong challenge. To see a 30 year old woman die on the operating table after having jumped in front of a train makes one wonder what was going on in her life that led her to do this. But it is also clear that while the physicians were working to save her, the need was to focus on the medical-surgical tasks confronting them. I could see that the young men who become paraplegic and quadraplegic as a result of motorcycle and water accidents need doctors who can help them with their medical needs and help them go on with their lives. But maybe doctors can also play a role in education for prevention.

I believe at this time that my interest lies in orthopedics. However, I am aware that much lies before me as I hope to start my medical education, and that I need the education, training and exposure to the full range of medicine, before making a lifelong commitment to a specialty.

Essay #26

My interest in medicine has developed over many years. As a child and adolescent, my parents and relatives filled our home with keen and insightful discussion of the profession. Both of my grandfathers were doctors, two of my uncles are cardiologists, and on one side of the family the tradition goes back four generations—when medicine could hardly claim to be a science.

The decision, however, to become a physician has developed in college as an ungentle fusion of my two majors: physics and English. I refrained from a conservative curriculum at the undergraduate level and this combination allowed me a full dose of the humanities and a strong foundation in the physical sciences.

While I continue to enjoy the abstract nature of these disiplines, I consider medicine the practical union of these academic interests: scientific procedures will produce undeniable results, and yet behind each physical ailment will be an individual with special needs and priorities. The double-edged nature of the health profession requires a divided perspective.

My summer work over the last several years further guided my interests in medicine. As a YMCA camp counselor, I gained great satisfaction working closely with others. Moreover, the importance of qualified medical attention and knowledge was driven home to me. As waterfront director, I taught Advanced Lifesaving to all the staff. One summer, one counselor dove into shallow water and injured his neck. A recently trained counselor recognized the cause of his friend's inactive prone position and carefully turned him over allowing him to breathe until the paramedics and doctor arrived to safely immobilize his neck.

Two summers ago, while working on a survey crew on a remote Navajo reservation in Arizona, I was fascinated by the need for culturally sensitive medical care. Good doctors there learned to explain their work and ask questions in ways that demonstrated an understanding of and a respect for a proud culture. Yet the need for primary care physicians was painfully obvious; the bubonic plague made its appearance several times that summer.

This past summer, I was privileged to work in West Germany with two renal physiologists, Dr. Beyenbach of Cornell University and Dr. Fromter of the Max Planck Institute. Earlier that year I had gained general lab experience working in Dr. Beyenback's lab at Cornell. Because of this experience, they allowed me to work quite independently to develop my own skills of physiological investigation.

Our main interest was ion specific channals present in the membranes of collecting duct cells in the mammalian kidney. To study channals, we employed the rather recent technique of patch clamp as developed by the German physiologist Neher. This technique uses tiny glass pipettes to electrically isolate small portions of a cell membrane. Channals can then be detected by the small currents that arise when ions of a specific polarity flow through the small pores of the membrane. I will present the results of this research this December at the American Society of Nephrology's Annual Meeting.

While my work this past summer proved by general abilities in research, I plan to practice medicine at the clinical level. Several factors influence this choice. First of all, I am a person of practical abilities. Although I often enjoy theoretical considerations, I consider myself to be most effective and useful dealing with individual problems. Secondly, I enjoy involvement with a variety of people and a variety of problems. Finally, I favor a more holistic approach in medicine, and toward that end I intend to practice primary-care medicine as a Family Practitioner.

Essay #27

A successful and effective physician must possess two essential qualities—a thirst for knowledge, and a deep motivation to aid his fellow man. Unfortunately, today's stereotypical "premed" student seems altogether preoccupied with the former at the exclusion of the latter. While a good doctor must possess an innate intelligence and an ability to expand and update his knowledge, it is equally important that he or she be able to effectively interact and communicate with the co-workers and patients that surround him. I believe my experiences and accomplishments at Cornell show that I possess both the necessary desire and essential skills needed to succeed in the field of medicine.

In satisfying my thirst for knowledge, I have pursued a broad range of courses and employment that demonstrate my raw abilities. Science has always fascinated me, and I think my academic choices reflect those interests. In addition, I have acted as a research assistant for the past two summers under Dr. Stefan Cohen of the University of Buffalo Department of Medicine at Buffalo General Hospital, examining the tumoricidal effects of isolated liver cells. My work culminated with the acceptance of a paper, which I coauthored, entitled "Augmentation of Natural Cytotoxicity of Murine Nonparenchymal Liver Cells by Interferon or Interleukin 2" for publication this fall in *Sinusoidal Liver Cells* by Elsevier Biomedical Press.

To be an informed participant in contemporary society, though, requires more than just scientific intelligence and rote memorization. To fully appreciate that being we call man, one must have experience in the informed reflection upon the literature, philosophy, and art of our society, as well as an understanding of politics, history, and economics. The broad range of academic and extracurricular activities I have pursued in college demonstrates my desire to gain an extremely comprehensive exposure to such material, as well as the skills to solve problems and process information.

But knowledge in and of itself is insufficient. I perceive knowledge not as an end, but as a means to an end—helping people. A simple glance at the activities I have participated in at Cornell clearly illustrates how crucial others are to me, and I think there is one obvious conclusion—I like people! Whether it's teaching, helping, entertaining, talking, or just enjoying a good laugh, I am comfortable, confident, and effective interacting with other people. I am a member of the Delta Chi fraternity, where I have acted as Alumni Secretary, Corresponding Secretary, and a member of the Executive Board. I have been quite active as a College Ambassador, hosting potential students and giving tours to visitors at Cornell. I have also acted as a student advisor, advising students on various aspects of Cornell— whether it be scheduling problems or just roommate trouble. On campus I've held a number of jobs, and have also acted as a teaching assistant for an Oral Communications class. In addition, I am presently acting as a TA for both an Animal Physiology Laboratory and a Microcomputer Applications course. Each of these activities requires not only a considerable amount of responsibility, but a good deal of patience as well.

By far the most enjoyable (and time consuming) activites I am involved in have been singing with the Cornell Glee Club, and a small men's *a cappella* subset called the HANGOVERS— known both for our singing and our sense of humor. In more than three years of activity, we have toured California, the South Eastern U.S. and various portions of the Northeast, released an album, and performed for numerous gatherings of students, alumni, and friends, as well as the likes of Helmut Schmidt, Henry Kissinger, Gerald Ford, and Bob Hope.

Clearly, I have not allowed myself to become trapped in the static environment of the "preprofessional" student. I have managed to both expand my scope of knowledge and grow as an individual. Yet throughout this whole process I have also managed to focus my interests and intensify my desires. Without hesitation, I can honestly say that there can be no better choice for me than a career in medicine, for medicine combines the best of both worlds—working closely with people while continuing in a scientific field. I firmly believe I have the ability to succeed in such a career, and will find great satisfaction in patient care. Through a career in medicine I can help man at his most basic level, his physical presence, and still grow individually while contributing to society's wealth of knowledge.

While intent on pursuing an active practice, possibly in pediatrics, orthopedics, oncology, or geriatrics, I fully intend to incorporate both clinical and experimental research into my work. Farther down the road, I would like to become involved in public policy as it relates to health care and science. It seems fairly obvious that governmental legislation and policy has lagged far behind the advances being made in many scientific fields, and needs to be updated. While active medical practice is my primary goal, I feel that I could contribute significantly to both the scientific community and the general public by acting as as advocate for science among the politicians.

Essay #28

Throughout the years I have spent in high school and college, my main career goal has been to become a physician. Although I have carefully examined many options, I feel that a career in medicine best suits my personal interests. Ever since I was a small child, I have had a special passion for biology. Understanding the various mechanisms and functions of the human body is my main biological interest. Through a thorough study and career in medicine, I believe that I will be able to satisfy my need to understand the various workings of the human system.

As a medical student and physician, I feel that I will be able to easily mix with the people who surround me. Being an only child (my 11-year old sister died when I was six years old), I was forced to interact with others in the community for social satisfaction. This enabled me to learn how to relate to a wide variety of people.

I have had a number of experiences with the medical profession, but my relationship with Dr. Henry Corn, a former family doctor now retired, sticks out most in my mind. Dr. Corn made patients feel at ease with his wit, humor, and compassion. His number one priority was the patient's health, and with this aspect, Dr. Corn was "strictly business." I feel that Dr. Corn was the epitome of the type of physician I will strive to be. It is important that doctors achieve a balance between subjectivity and objectivity. Through my experience observing Dr. Corn, I saw that he was a master at expressing proper concern for his patients, while not letting his concern get in the way of sound professional judgment.

Another person who has been a special influence to me is Herbert Hantz, my high-school English teacher. Mr. Hantz worked with me many times before and after school, teaching the importance of written expression as a complement to speech communication. He also instilled in me that there is honor and dignity in working hard to achieve goals. Even now, I call on Mr. Hantz from time to time to receive profitable advice and counsel.

During the summer before my first year of college, I had the opportunity to travel through Europe on a study tour with about thirty of my high-school classmates. In thirty-one days we traveled through the countries of Germany, Switzerland, Italy, France and England. This was the first time in my life that I met so many different people with varying cultural backgrounds. The trip helped me alleviate much of my ignorance about the world beyond America. Through socializing with the Europeans of differing countries, I learned the basic lesson that people are people wherever you go. Although there are many differences between the citizens of the world, we are all human beings experiencing joy, pain, anger and sorrow.

My commitment to medicine will be the largest factor affecting my success in the field. I have put a great deal of time and energy into seeking a medical career. Once this goal is obtained, my persistance will not subside. I feel that a physician is a public servant, one who must take the responsibility of giving that "extra effort" to insure that a patient gets the best medical care possible.

I firmly believe that I will make a viable contribution to the medical school to which I am accepted. I have the strength to carry on when the workload gets tough, and I also have the perseverence to weather setbacks that I will face. The school that accepts me will receive an excited student who will prove to the board of admissions that they did not make a mistake.

Essay #29

It has been my ambition, for some time, to become involved in the medical profession. I chose medicine because I feel it is my duty in life to concern myself with the well being of others. This duty can best be fulfilled to my satisfaction by pursuing a career in medicine.

To fulfill my aspirations there are certain key qualities that I must acquire. I have begun to prepare for that responsibility by maintaining a strong academic background and involving myself in extracurricular activities and clinical experiences.

My undergraduate education has provided a strong background for my future studies in medical school. With a B.S. in Microbiology, I have acquired an indepth knowledge of the biological sciences. I have been able to improve my research and scientific skills by applying the knowledge to my Microbiology lab work with pathogenic organisms, such as *Neisseria gonnorhoae.*

The life of a good, dedicated physician involves more than knowing how the body functions. Equally important, is knowing how to deal with people on a personal basis. I have acquired some clinical experience in the area of interpersonal relationships. Two years ago I volunteered as a nurses aid at a local hospital. I worked primarily with elderly patients and became more sensitive to their special needs. This summer I am working as a volunteer in an Emergency Room. This experience has given me the opportunity to observe doctors and nurses in critical situations. I am also working with a doctor in his private practice. My duties involve filing charts, assisting patients, urine and stool analysis and developing X rays. I feel these experiences are invaluable to me in developing a sensitivity to patients and their needs.

My ethnic background has been a contributing factor in my prospective plan after medical school. I would like to work in a physician shortage area where a Puerto Rican background will be helpful in dealing with other hispanic minorities.

I want to succeed in my career goals. I will be a successful doctor if I am able to give the sick the compassion and quality medical care that they deserve.

Essay #30

Simply stated, childhood accidents and subsequent visits to pediatricians, dentists, and hospitals established my interest in medicine. During these sessions, I was slowly exposed to many disciplines of practical medicine—radiology, anesthesiology, thoracic surgery, plastic surgery, emergency room medicine, and orthopedics. Although the visits themselves were not unusual for an active child, my enthusiasm may have been so; a broken bone presented another chance to see "how doctors worked".

As I grew, so did my enthusiasm for medicine. Fortunately, this fervor also matured. To my delight, I found that I didn't have to break an arm or step on a rusty nail to learn a little bit more about medicine. I turned rather to books, magazines, journals, and other sources of information. Very quickly, it was clear that medicine was not just doctors and hospitals but that it pervaded society in a very broad sense. With that realization, I began a scholastic, physical, and emotional approach to an eventual career in medicine.

During the second half of my freshman year at the University of Michigan, I applied for and was awarded a competitive pre-medical/medical scholarship through the United States Air Force. A part of this application required me to write a tentative plan of study for the following undergraduate years. This outline has served as the basis for my directed liberal-arts education. My studies have included subjects from molecular biology to astronomy and from comparative politics to the literature of Thomas Mann. This Summer, I have supplemented these studies with practical laboratory experience both full-time in immunology under Dr. Latham Claflin and on a volunteer basis in Dr. Benedict Lucchesi's pharmacology laboratory.

Because I am most mentally fit when I am physically fit, my undergraduate years have also included a host of recreational and competitive sports. Regular tennis and squash matches as well as seasonal competition on the University of Michigan Rowing Team, therefore, have also contributed to my approach toward medicine.

Emotionally, there are both planned and unplanned events which prepare me for that side of medicine. Among those planned are challenging academic schedules as well as a year of study in Freiburg, West Germany. Occasionally, each of these examples was a source of stress and anxiety to be overcome. Planned psychological challenges, however, are often dwarfed by those not forecast. For many years, my father struggled to live with bipolar affective disorder and schizophrenia. As a family, we struggled with him. Last August, however, we had to involuntarily hospitalize him. He has since left our family. As the oldest of four children, I have been faced with both the loss of my father and a redefining of my role in the family. The events of this last year have caused me to question nearly everything I had taken for granted and have made me aware of unsuspected reservoirs of strength I had not known before.

I view my eventual career in medicine as one filled with both sacrifice and intangible reward. From broken bones and stepped-on rusty nails to directed collegiate years and unforseen tragedy, I have followed a pathway toward these sacrifices and gains. With all of the experiences which have prepared me for events to come, I anticipate four years of medical school with enthusiasm.

Essay #31

The greatest motivational factor in my pursuit of a medical career was my work experience with the DuPont Company in the Cornell Engineering Co-Op Program. The seven months of research I performed at DuPont impressed upon me the similarities between my Chemical Engineering background and the increasingly technical nature of medicine. I was a member of a research group actively involved in improving certain types of polymers for industrial, as well as medical, applications. Polymers of this type find use in medicine due to their inert properties in the human body and other biological environments. As a research engineer, I also had the opportunity to learn about innovations within DuPont's Biomedical Products research laboratories. Here, I became aware of improvements in biotechnology and computers that will inevitably have a significant impact upon the quality of health care. Through this work experience in the engineering field, however, I also recognized that I wanted a career which places a greater emphasis on human relationships. A career in medicine will allow me to work with and help people in a more direct manner than I found possible in my engineering work.

As a student at Cornell University, I received a broad exposure to a variety of scientific disciplines which are the basis of many of today's rapidly advancing medical technologies. My interests in organic chemistry, biochemistry, and the engineering sciences were particularly important in forming my decision to enter a health-related career. I consider medicine to be a means for me to apply these or similar sciences in a most fulfilling and humane manner. In addition, I believe that the practical nature of my engineering education has afforded me a superior problem-solving ability that can be applied to medicine as well as other scientific fields.

After my formal education at Cornell, it was my intention to work two years in the engineering profession before entering medical school. During this time, I hoped to gain practical skills and management experience relevant to my future medical career. I worked for the Nestle Company following graduation as a manager-in-training in their food processing operations. At Nestle, I learned about the nutritional aspects of health and worked with people in my role as a supervisor.

After nine months with Nestle, I decided to accept another management position in mechanical design and manufacturing with the Ulster Tool and Die Corporation in Kingston, N.Y. My technical work at this firm, designing and developing specialized machinery, has given me the valuable knowledge of how people interact with mechanical devices. More importantly though, this opportunity to manage people in a professional environment has proven to be a most challenging and enjoyable task, confirming my decision to pursue a health career. The consistently high level of performance expected of me as a manager and engineer in this business has been an excellent preparation for my future responsibilities as a physician.

While being employed by Ulster Tool and Die, I have been performing volunteer work in the Radiology Department of the Benedictine Hospital in Kingston, N.Y. My work here, transporting and assisting patients for testing, has increased my familiarity with hospital procedures and proven to be a personally rewarding experience for me. From these practical pursuits in the hospital, working directly with patients and observing firsthand the realities of hospital life, I have had a candid introduction to health careers.

These varied experiences have given me the opportunity to more clearly define my professional goals. The time I have spent since my graduation from Cornell has been particularly important to me for personal growth and for making a more informed decision towards medicine. My strong background in the basic sciences, and the practical work experience I have in both the chemical industry and the hospital, have motivated me to pursue a health career.

To fulfill the medical school requirements, I completed the Biology requirement during the Summer of 1984 at Pace University. In order to accommodate the work schedule for the Cornell Engineering Co-Op Program, I completed the Fall 1982 semester's courses during the Summer of 1982. I worked for DuPont during the Fall of 1982 and the Summer of 1983. My participation in the Cornell Engineering Co-Op Program necessitated that I fulfill the organic chemistry requirement with the following sequence of courses: Organic Chemistry 253 (4 credit hours), Experimental Organic Chem. 251 (2 credit hours), and Industrial Organic Processes 421 (2 credit hours).

Essay #32

I was born Dutch and spent the first nine years of my life in the Netherlands. At that time my father retired and took the family to France. We lived for fourteen years on the Swiss-French border outside of Geneva. The international atmosphere of Geneva was represented by the children at the International School of Geneva, where I was a student through high school. For example, one unique experience during high school was participating in the "Student United Nations". For three days students from several European schools acted as diplomats from the countries represented at the United Nations. The exposure and sharing of the varied culture, religions, traditions and languages has continued to help me to accept people for what they are and to be able to adjust more readily to diverse situations. By maintaining a certain level of academic achievement I was permitted to participate in sports. I enjoyed being a member of many teams especially, ski, basketball and track teams. I felt honored to be named sports woman of the year during my senior year. Although all sports brought me pleasure, skiing was my favorite. Therefore, I pursued it more intensely and eventually raced for the Dutch National ski team. At this level, skiing was demanding not only physically but also mentally. My memories of the pressure, losing as well as winning, but especially the comradery will always remain with me.

After high school I decided to continue my education at the University of Geneva. I had three particular interests, people, nature and sciences. Medicine was a serious consideration but due to the conservative attitude of my parents and Switzerland, the idea of a woman in medicine was not well supported. Without the obvious role models to look up to, I chose to study Biology. The University was rather academically oriented without emphasis on athletic or social activities. Nonetheless, I felt compelled to continue to compete in basketball, sailing and skiing. My last year of the University was spent involved in an independent research project in microbiology. The results of which were the basis of my thesis entitled "Analysis of the genetic polymorphism of the HLA-DRB genes coding for class II antigenes of the human histocompatibility complex". The research was fascinating and challenging but on the other hand I realized it was not as idealistic as I had imagined it to be. I liked the technology and knowledge involved in basic science but I found myself missing a more direct interaction with people.

That same year in the laboratory, I met the most wonderful man in the world who is now my husband. Mark was a Fulbright Scholar from the United States doing a year of research in Geneva. Fortunately, I completed my studies at the same time Mark finished his research. Therefore, I was able to go with Mark to the United States in August 1983 when he started at Cornell Medical School. It was my first time in the United States and the transition was made easier by Mark, his family and the fact that two of my best friends from high school happened to live in New York at the time. Since I was not yet a permanent resident it was initially difficult to find a job. After several waitressing jobs, a cardiologist hired me as his secreatary. It was all new to me but I enjoyed the work, especially the patient contact. The atmosphere revived my old interest in medicine and I decided to continue my education. Again I considered medical school, but the surgical assistant program seemed like a perfect compromise. Being newly married a particular concern of mine was having the time for a family in the future. A shorter education with some responsibility and patient contact made the role of a surgical assistant look ideal. I loved learning about the applications of science in medicine, mastering some surgical techniques, and especially my interaction with the patients on the wards. Unfortunately, I soon realized that our short didactic course led us to become more technically oriented rather than problem solving members of the surgical team. I finally decided that I would never feel comfortable in this situation and that being an assistant would never satisfy me. Therefore, I quit the program to reevaluate my future plans.

This was not terribly difficult. By now I had had more exposure to the demands of medicine, what medicine represents, and had spent some time discussing the issues of women in medicine. Therefore, I now feel comfortable and excited about becoming a physician. So, with the support of Mark, I decided to pursue what deep inside I always wanted to do, apply for medical school.

Essay #33

What kind of person would be insane enough to spend half of his life studying for a job which requires twelve hour work days, no vacations, and interminable patience — in other words total dedication? He must be a person who realizes the many responsibilities which such a prestigious, yet taxing vocation will require. Also, he must have observed the pride which a doctor feels when his patient is no longer dependent on others. I am such a person.

As a child, I was asthmatic. Though this never kept me from my daily romps through the mud on the way to school or from relishing every moment of gym class, I sometimes became ill at night. No matter what the hour, Dr. Orange would always come to the rescue, with a bag of medicine and a box of soothing words. Dr. Orange was my champion and I vowed to some day follow in his footsteps. This news was received enthusiastically by my parents who always encouraged my academic interests. Thus began my quest to become the first doctor in my family.

Although almost all of my hopes and dreams have changed since childhood, my longing to become a doctor has stood fast. My experience working at the Stanford VA Hospital has been a major force in solidifying this desire. I have been working in a psychopharmacology lab there for the past three years. I am very lucky to be a part of a lab in which I am treated as an equal with all other personnel, doctors, and researchers. I have become good friends with many of the doctors with whom I work. Whether it is during a three hundred tube assay or during a day of champagne tasting, I have seen the true life of a physician through the eyes of those who know: the politics involved, the hard work, and the great stress. Yet, I am a person who thrives on new and exciting challenges, and the thought of hard work does not have a negative connotation.

My own research has a taught me quite a lot as well. I am currently concluding my Human Biology honors project which I have been working on for the past year and am confident will be published this fall. It involves my testing the neurochemical and behavioral effects of a new drug, called Proglumide, to determine whether it can be used to treat Schizophrenia. Through this project I have learned to work on my own, solving problems which arose at the most inopportune times. I have become aware of the wealth of knowledge which one can acquire through hands on experience and by conversation with fellow research enthusiasts. I have experienced the humiliation and sense of helplessness one feels when an assay just will not work. Yet, I have also known the feeling of an incredible high when my first paper was published. I regard my research experience as one of the highlights of my undergraduate career. However, I like working with people, and I hope to experience the clinical side of medicine during my years in medical school; this will afford me the opportunity to decide exactly where I wish to put my energies during my years as a doctor.

What kind of person would go into medicine? A person who can endure the hardships in the hopes that one day he will hear the words, "Thanks Doc" from a patient who, a few hours earlier, could hardly breath, no less talk.

Essay #34

My activities at Cornell and in the Ithaca-Cayuga Heights communities are not preparations or exercises for a future way of life but are my way of life. Community service and working with people have always stimulated my daily experiences and have made my life more meaningful. The desire to make people's lives more tolerable and a penchant for scientific research are two qualities that can best be combined in a career in medicine. Thus, my motivations lie in the firm belief that I can make a considerable change in the human condition — for the better.

My medically related experience has been three-fold: volunteer hospital work, medical science research and ambulance service. First, at Bellevue, I worked in the Tumor Registry as the one responsible for interpreting patients' records and staging diagnosed cases of cancer. Although this was not a clinical experience, I learned a great deal of pathology, anatomy and medical terminology. I was also allowed to participate in Residents' discussions in the Ob.-Gyn. department next door where I became temporarily proficient at recognizing neoplastic cells and staging the endometrium from slides. This same summer, on alternate days, I volunteered as a research assistant, assisting a study on the pathology of cerebral brain ischemia in rats. This experience enabled me to sharpen my laboratory skills and understand the problems associated with medical research. Second, the next summer I conducted my own study investigating the lipid peroxide content of various foods under the supervision of M.L. Seligman, Ph.D. and H.B. Demopolous, M.D. (Klausner et al., J. Cornell Scientists, 1:1 and submitted J. Food Science). This study taught me about the value of preventative medicine, forced me to apply my knowledge of organic chemistry and familiarized me with the entire design of medical research from the conception of an idea to the publishing of the results. Third, I am a N.Y. State Certified Emergency Medical Technician and have served on a volunteer ambulance corps since 1980 and a rescue squad since 1983. These trauma experiences have been invaluable training for a career in medicine. I have learned how to stabilize patients through basic procedures and equally important how to inspire confidence in my coworkers.

My volunteer work with the Tompkins County 4-H includes

organizing weekly activities for a group of teenagers from the ages of 14-19. I use my Planned Parenthood training to educate them in contraception and offer frank sexual advice. I find this experience very rewarding and a welcome relief from the pressures at Cornell.

Being a member of Phi Kappa Sigma Fraternity has allowed me to exercise my great leadership and motivational abilities. The office of President gave me a chance to change the attitude and reputation of the Chapter from one of complacency and disorganization to activism and efficiency. Under my direction as Rush Chairman we were able to increase our new membership from an abysmal one in 1983-4 to eight in 1984-85 and I have been re-elected to this position for Fall 1985.

Perhaps my most interesting, at least my newest endeavor, was the creation and publication of the Journal of Cornell Scientists. I realized a lack of opportunities existed for undergradutes to publish research where their peers could read it and they could practice the format of scientific publication. The remedy was simple: to create such a journal on my own; however, the process was difficult and took a lot of ingenuity, Funds needed to be raised, a publisher found and submissions acquired. Within three months of the inception of the idea all three facets were readily realized and the first issue appeared in November, 1984.

The varied activities that I pursue indicate that I am a determined, motivated and conscientious individual, all essential qualities for a career in medicine. I perform well under pressure as any fellow firefighter will attest and get along remarkably well with youngsters, peers and elders. My future plans include incorporating my concern for human welfare, creativity and leadership abilities in becoming a surgeon, researcher and public policy official.

Essay #35

During my years at Manhattan College, I have become determined in my desire to pursue a career in medicine. Condfident of my abilities and determination, I sincerely believe I possess the qualities to become a caring physician. Aside from academic achievement, I have demonstrated leadership qualities, intiative and an ability to empathize and to communicate with people.

At Manhattan College I chose to study electrical engineering because its stringent science curriculum would allow me to branch into other career fields. In my studies I have become aware of the many applications of electronic devices in medicine and I would like to apply my engineering education with a medical education to enable me to research and design or improve medical equipment. In order to learn more about medical application of electrical engineering, I have registered for a biomedical engineering course and am currently participating in a Manhattan College senior project in conjunction with the Orthontics and Prosthetics Department of New York University Medical Center designing electric circuitry to improve the N.Y.U. Hosmer Prosthetic Elbow.

As a member of Eta Kappa Nu, National Honor Society of Electrical Engineers, I served as a tutor for other electrical engineering students and participated in the design, construction and presentation of an electrical stimulator to reduce muscle pain for Manhattan College Open House ceremonies. I was selected to New York Zi Chapter of Tau Beta Pi, National Engineering Honor Society, and am currently serving on the chapter Executive Board and selection committee and represent the chapter at district events.

At Manhattan College I served as a group leader in the Freshman Orientation Program. Later, I was selected to serve in their Peer Counselor Program in which upper classmen offer peer assistance and direction to freshman through the semester, beginning with general orientation and including weekly group meetings and work-shops on study habits and test anxiety. Since freshman year, I have been an active member of Alpha Phi Delta National Fraternity, serving as a member of the Judiciary Committee, Intramural Chairman, Pledgemaster and chapter organization. I have helped organize and have participated in many charity fund raising events for organizations such as the American Heart Association, Special Olympics and the American Cancer Society and have also participated in a program with the Methodist Church Home for the Aged, spending time with the elderly people at the home. The ability to communicate and work with others has been an essential element of much of my activities at Manhattan College.

For the past seven years I have worked at Carvel Ice Cream Store No. 699 on Staten Island and have served as a weekend and night manager for the past four years. The money I have earned together with my scholarship and student loan has helped pay for my college expenses. In the summer following my sophomore year, I volunteered in the emergency room of Bayley Seton Hospital on Staten Island. This enabled me to observe medical professionals at work and to understand the dedication and teamwork necessary for successful patient care.

I recognize that many factors must be considered in choosing medical students. I am confident that my background in academics, extracurricular activities, community involvement and personal commitment fulfill the qualifications you seek in applicants.

Essay #36

I have always been interested in science and have practiced studio art and have wrestled for ten years. But it is difficult to expain my interest in three such widely differing pursuits as part of an underlying state of mind. After some thought, I was surprised to realize that there is indeed a similar motivation for all three activities.

This motivation relates to a deep interest I have always had in mythology and science fiction. The stories that most appeal to me are of individuals alienated from, or cast into, an alien society, struggling to assert their independence and individuality. By suspending my disbelief, I can partake in the struggle of the fictional characters and feel their victories and defeats. Art, wrestling and science are all, in a sense, isolating activities, and each requires a great deal of discipline and training. One cannot paint a picture the first time one steps into a studio; nor can one wrestle well the first time on a mat. Research requires the patience to gather the proper data, and also creativity to interpret the data correctly. These three interests have served as my way of becoming in reality the adventurers I have read about.

Let me elaborate. Several months ago, I was busy writing my thesis. I have already spent the better part of a year gathering data and running assays in a laboratory, and all that was left was the interpretation of the data. I found that instead of dreading the long hours of writing and rewriting, I looked forward to it. I felt that I was fitting in the final pieces of a large jigsaw puzzle or coming to the end of an intricate detective story, and it was exciting to watch the overall picture slowly emerge. The feeling, surprisingly, was akin to a feeling I often get whenever I draw an excellent picture or wrestle a perfect match. In all these instances, I achieve a certain rhythm and feeling of inspiration that enables me to work with a minimum of energy. It is said that long distance runners experience a feeling called "runners' high," that makes them addicted to their running. The high I experience when I wrestle and win a match, draw an excellent picture or piece together bits of research is just as addictive. When I read science fiction, I identify with the protagonist because I feel that the control and effort vital to their successes are similar to qualities in myself that enable me to spend ten hours straight working on a picture, or spend weeks preparing for a wrestling match.

I have always wanted to be a doctor because I have sensed that much of a doctor's work will satisfy me in the way that my other interests satisfy me. I am careful, however, not to confuse my love of adventure and fantasy with my reasons for wanting to be a physician. For a long time I had conceived of myself as going through the medical training process so that I could become a "doctor/hero." Wielding a shining scalpel, I would cure all of my patients' problems with stunning success. What I now realize is that for most of my future patients, there will be no one sure method of treatment, and many of them may not respond to treatment at all.

Thus, it is my feeling that a doctor should be more than a dispenser of health care; he should also take an active role in the health community. It seems to me that the rising cost of health care and increasingly bewildering technology have created a breach in the rapport between doctors and the public. Many patients feel that they have little control or understanding of their treatment. As a doctor, I may not be able to cure or even help all of my patients, but, if I can help to bridge the gap between my and my patients' knowledge, then I will be as satisfied as I ever was reading myths and fiction. When I am a physician, I feel that the discipline and control I have learned from my other interests will serve me well, but more importantly I feel that the enthusiasm and joy that I derive from these interests will also be an internal part of my life as a doctor. Hopefully, my future patients will sense my enthusiasm and be encouraged by it.

Essay #37

Although I have learned a great deal through formal course work, this has provided only a part of my education. During the past year, I have had the opportunity to work in an operating room (Summer '84) and an emergency room (Winter '84- Spring '85) of hospitals at home and at college. Although quite different, both were valuable learning experiences. In the operating room, I was able to observe how the hospital staff worked together in performing the mechanics of an operation. The emergency room, on the other hand, allowed me to see the impact that illness had on the patient and those close to him. These experiences have taught me that in addition to mastering the technical skills, success is dependent on the personal qualities of the physician. These qualities include compassion, emotional strength, and the ability to instill confidence in people.

I have developed some of these personal qualities in my work as a camp counselor for underprivileged children (Summer '83) and as a Big Brother (1983-84) to a young boy living near my college. These experiences have also allowed me to know the feeling of having people depend on me, which is an important aspect of being a physician.

This summer I am working in a laboratory at The Sloan-Kettering Cancer Institute. I have always had a strong interest in research. I believe that investigative work helps build an inquiring, independent, and analytical approach to learning while developing the ability to evaluate and solve problems with ingenuity. The rapid therapeutic advances of today make this an asset, not only in academic careers such as medical research and teaching, but in clinical practice as well.

My parents are physicians so I have always been exposed to the field of medicine, a field which has interested me for much of my life. The past few years have provided opportunities for me to test this interest and strengthen my decision to pursue a career in medicine. It is a career which I am confident will provide numerous challenges and a lifetime of learning.

Essay #38

As a person who is highly interested in the sciences and in people, a career in medicine has always appealed to me. The ability to heal the sick is a gift I hope to attain and put to use. As time passes, I am more eager to become a surgeon and to practice medicine in or near a large city.

My first medical related experience occurred in the summer after my sophomore year of high school. I participated in the American Foundation for Negro Affairs Program (AFNA). This program supported the idea that more minorities were needed in the medical profession and financed tours of medical schools, showed filmstrips of surgical procedures, and presented lectures by medical doctors. AFNA increased my interest in medicine tremendously and was a major influence in my decision to become a doctor.

During my junior year, I became a volunteer worker at Lafon Nursing Home in New Orleans where I worked closely with the nurses and residents. This not only required me to learn several duties of nursing, but also taught me to become patient, understanding, and perservering in dealing with others.

The following summer I attended the Stress on Analytical Reasoning Program (SOAR) at Xavier University. Its purpose is to prepare incoming students for science and math courses. This program was the final determining factor in my becoming a Chemistry major at Xavier University.

In the sumer of 1982, prior to entering Xavier, I became a volunteer worker at Louisiana State Medical School in New Orleans. As a result, I participated in research studies pertaining to cancer as an inherited disease. In addition, I actively participated in the growth of amniotic fluid cell cultures which helped me to learn the importance of cleanliness and sterile equipment.

At Xavier, I am a member of various social organizations and academic honor socities. At the end of my sophomore year, a decision was made to become less involved in extracurricular activities and to focus my energies on my courses. As a result, I completed the junior year, my hardest year as a Chemistry major, even more motivated than before. The science courses that I have taken left me fascinated with the structure and systems of the human body. I wish to continue my quest for knowledge in medical school, to further my understanding of how the body functions.

While attending Xavier, I also held a job as a student lab assistant in the hematology department of Charity Hospital in New Orleans. For two years I worked approximately twenty-five hours a week and became very familiar with the operations of this department. I tested blood for sickle cell anemia and learned how to do retic counts, but became most experienced in urinalysis. In addition, I was able to see how doctors are viewed by other hospital personnel.

Intrinsically, I am highly motivated. Extrinsically, I have a loving supportive family and the confidence of the highly competent faculty of Xavier. Together, the above supply me with the confidence, courage and knowledge needed not only to attend medical school, but also to succeed. Having spent the last several years of life preparing to learn how to help the sick and the needy, I feel that my talents can best be exercised by becoming a doctor and working to heal others. This is my goal in life.

Essay #39

As a child I believed that the answer to the polite old question of what would I like to do when I grow-up was a simple one. One just chose what one did best, most naturally and loved the most. It seemed so easy to answer; I would grow-up and help people. Although my basic approach had a lot of truth to it, my naivete of the complexities of decision-making is apparent. Knowledgeable decisions require more than just good instinct.

All the truly important resolutions in our lives require time and care. Benjamin Franklin used to sit and write out the pros and cons of each problem before arriving at a decision. He gave each reason a rating which he then tallied for an answer carrying the highest score. This process gave him the opportunity to identify the really weighty issues and allowed him to take the wisest course.

As a thoughtful individual I can appreciate Franklin's approach as I have come to live the pros and cons which have led me to my recent career-decision. My desire to study medicine was born out of my attempts to understand and help people and my pursuit of the discipline of psychology.

I have studied many perspectives in psychology and the more I learned the more I realized that the field had too narrow a focus on people. It really addressed only half the issue of human development by virtually ignoring the biological aspects of human behavior. Understanding the whole individual means learning about both the psychological and biological facets since neither is complete without the other. Having recognized this vital link between the two fields, I have actively dedicated myself to pursuing a career that encompasses both disciplines.

I have never let go of my interest in people. To really excel and truly appreciate my career choice, I have held on to my youthful ideal of identifying with that special quality of helping people which comes so naturally to me. While some would be reluctant to change course, I have welcomed the challenge and allowed my experience in psychology to help me clearly define my goals. I, unfortunately, took chemistry at a time when it had little relevance in my life; psychology had consumed my interest. I missed most of the classes and should have dropped the course; a mistake that I hope is one of very few.

By taking the time to explore and better organize my skills, I have also been able to make a knowledgeable and intellectually sound decision.

Essay #40

Some of my foremost objectives in the past three years have been to obtain a "well rounded" education, determine the benefits of a medical career, and to prepare myself adequately for such a career. By choosing a social science (economics) as a major and by working in research labs at the University of Minnesota (Minneapolis) Medical School during the past three summers, I believe I have attained all three goals. My transcript and recommendations attest my progress in the first goal. In the remaining essay, I will comment on my progress in the latter two.

Having witnessed a limited sample of the routines of physicians at the University of Minnesota hospital during the past three summers, I think one of the greatest satisfactions of practicing medicine would be correctly diagnosing a patient, prescribing an effective treatment, and observing the patient's recovery. Moreover, a physician would be able to reap these benefits daily.

In the long run though, I would like to be a physician who researches medicine on a "basic science" level and, at the same time, translates advances in scientific theory into clinical practice. I have spent the past two summers working on projects which, at first, do not appear applicable to current medical problems, but may eventually help lead to new clinical treatments. For example, last summer I researched the effects of human fibrinogen on the phagocytosis of *Escherichia coli* by human polymorphonuclear neutrophils (PMNs). My study revealed that an indirect relationship exists between fibrinogen concentration and phagocytic killing by neutrophils. This conclusion might appear interesting but clinically of little value; it may, however, help elucidate the mechanism by which fibrin clots inhibit phagocytosis of *E. coli* by neutrophils. Hence, a treatment could be developed which might prevent the formation of peritoneal abscesses and intraabdominal sepsis. An accomplishment like this would be, I believe, of great and lasting satisfaction.

Presently, I am working on a project studying the effects of hyperoxia on cutaneous wounds. The literature reveals that when an inoculum of *E. coli* is injected intradermally with a mass inoculation gun into a guinea pig, the resultant lesion will be smaller if the animal is contained in a hyperoxic environment. The literature, so far, makes no reference to a mechanism. To identify this mechanism is the object of my current investigation.

The research hypothesis loosely reads, "increased partial pressures of oxygen in the ambient air lead to a more effective exidative burst on the part of the neutrophils; thus, bacteria are cleared from the wound more quickly, and the wound can heal faster." The practical applications of this project are more readily apparent than in my previous research. People with cutaneous wounds could be treated more effectively with the administration of oxygen. Again, an advancement in the understanding of a basic science problem, such as wound healing, would have been translated into clinical practice. Satisfactions such as this are one of my main reasons for choosing medicine.

Essay #41

Praeludium. In the beginning there was dissonnance. The lifeless world was still and silent. Then God breathed life unto man, giving realm of his own. And then one night, man was given the power to create, to discover and to question. And as he created fire to heal him from the cold he discovered the sound of the flickers generated by his fire-maker. Like Apollo's Lyre when forged by Hermes, man's instrument was imbued with the magic of life. The magic to heal him from the cold he called medicine. The magic to create new sounds which brought him internal warmth he called music . . . Undoubtedly, music and medicine were born on the same day. From Apollo, who is god of both, to Johannes Brahms' best friend and trusted critic, the famous surgeon Theodore Billroth, music and medicine have courted each other incessantly. I am in love with both.

Allegro ma non troppo. My love for music is more than the desire to compose, interpret and listen; like my love for medicine is more than the desire to conduct research, practice and study. Rather, I wish to understand these two worlds, to internalize their principles so they become second nature to me, for love alone is not enough. I have not always felt this way: I decided to pursue medicine only after my second year in college. And music was not very exciting to me when I was sixteen. Unrelated yet similar incidents propelled me into these realms. I don't really know how it happened, but one day while playing the piano, I decided to improvise. As I played new combinations of notes, I felt free, uninhibited. Needless to say my improvisations soon became compositions. Discovering that I could be original, treading on my own musical road was one of the greatest gifts of life, because it radically modified my approach to music. In medicine it happened differently. During my first 2 years in college I wished to become a biochemical researcher, but a key factor unknown to me was missing. During spring break I volunteered to do social work in a small Mexican village. With some romanticism I observed the village physician work with his rudimentary instrumentation healing, teaching and mainly learning in this isolated Shangri-La. Like with music, I learned that this physician could heal in his own creative way and be rich in spite of this town's emptiness. Doing this required creativity and openness. However I made many mistakes after that because I asked what if . . . I only compose? What if I study only medicine?

Andante. Soon after beginning to compose, my piano skills were weakened and I found myself lacking discipline. Eventually, my composition ceased because there was no knowledge on which to base my ideas. Similarly, I began to doubt my studies at Stanford. It seemed so much easier to return to Mexico where one begins medical school after high school . . . In music and medicine there exists a fine artistic domain which permits individual expression, care and much subjectivity. Yet this freedom can subsist because there is a rigid framework supporting and fueling it. To the composer this freedom is the realm of emotions. In the medical world this artistic domain is expressed in the individuality of each person. Often, even in what appears to be straight procedural medicine, one finds room for subjectivity. I once translated for a urologist with a Spanish—speaking patient. She had been preliminarily diagnosed with kidney stones and came to see a specialist. The urologist began with an interview rather than a physical. As he progressed he soon discovered that the patient's husband was abusing her both sexually and physically. No kidney stones were found and she was subsequently treated by a therapist. I was inspired by this physician's ability to seek alternate explanations, literally outside his area of expertise. But he was able to carry this freedom because his understanding of medicine is so complete, and so profound. So I decided to study harmony and develop a deeper understanding of music. It then became evident to me that Stanford was the right choice. Perhaps the common bond between music and medicine is their dual nature. There seems to be no clear border between the artistic and the scientific aspects of either. The famous composer Shoenberg once said that everything of supreme value in art must show "heart" as well as "brain". Perhaps this is the most important lesson I have learned: to use my subjective freedom better by strengthening its fundamental base. When I began my research on eating disorders I was given much freedom, being able to design studies entirely by myself. The only given was the issue to address. At that point I began to cherish the vast resources of the medical library, in strengthening my knowledge. In music, when I began to play the flute, I decided to focus on technique rather than feeling. And I have learned more about both in the last year, than ever before. With the flute I have also discovered the joys of multi-instrumental music, chamber music. The ideal medical team should be like a chamber ensemble, each contributing to the whole, yet not drowning the others or becoming impersonal. I would like to practice thus.

Adagio. Important as music is to me, I have not considered music vocationally. Mainly for one reason: even though I love to perform, and write music for others, music plays a selfish role in my life. It challenges my senses and intelligence, and often it heals me, yet I cannot offer my knowledge to others. Medicine offers me many of the same challenges and satisfactions that music does, yet throughout I know that I can act for others as well. This is vital to me. In the past few weeks I have suffered because of the earthquake in my Mexico City. That day, especially, there was no room for music, only for medicine and I grieved for my lack of knowledge.

Allegro con spirite. Whenever I study a musical piece I study the biography of the composer. I believe that music always reflects the personality of the composer. Sometimes it reflects temporal feelings; others it reflects the composer's constant views on life. I choose to believe this because my music is entirely human. I write music for people, and sometimes write about people; but I always write as a human. In the same way I choose to believe that medicine is primarily human. It is very easy to lose track of this, especially while doing research, when one thinks in terms of enzymes and tRNA. I like to see both music and medicine in "Gestalt" terms. As I face my instrument, myriads of combinations flash across my mind and I visualize the harmonic implications of many, yet I cannot explain how I piece my notes together. Something deeper which I know not is ever present in my style. In medical terms, I've observed this in Anorexia Nervosa. This disorder is treated by some with pure psychology, others treat it as a physiological sickness. Yet there's much more to it. On one level there exists social pressure, family problems etc.; but deeper there must be a physiological mechanism which operates concurrently with the rest. One world influences the other resulting in a deadlocked circle. Subtle feelings which permeate my harmony, of the subtle biochemical processes that transcend the purely psychological; always knowing that this is life I am dealing with. Music and medicine have no lives of their own. Man gives them life so that they might celebrate his life. My flute lies before me, inorganic, not even latent. And yet I breathe life unto it and it speaks, sings, soothes. So lies my profession before me, and I can hardly wait to breathe life unto it so that it may in turn speak, sing, soothe and heal, breathing new life unto others.

Essay #42

Senior year at The Spence School, I discovered how inter-related the sciences could be. Understanding the basis of computer function and its similarities to the electrochemical nature of the nervous system, I realized how interesting the study of nature would be, especially with regards to the human system.

The summer following graduation I worked in the lab of Dr. P. R. Smith studying protein structure through electron microscopy. I was amazed how such research was based on basic principles within my grasp. I also began to realize how research on a day-to-day basis evolves rather than explodes, progressing by a series of smaller steps and variations on known procedures. The entire process seemed more like creative "playing" than work, despite the vast amount of knowledge behind each new variation. For two summers I worked in this lab developing a procedure to record electron micrographs of rotated crystals making possible 3-D reconstruction of the protein.

The following two summers I worked for Dr. Robert D. Allen at the Marine Biological Laboratory in Woods Hole. Dr. Allen was a role model in both professional and personal aspects. In the lab Dr. Allen had perfected the art of "playing" with a specimen and allowed me free rein to do the same. It was here I learned the value of "playing" with a specimen (in educated ways) in order to obtain the desired result. Our attempts to disturb the microtubules in extruded axoplasm resulted in our paper on "gliding microtubules" (1985). Outside the lab Dr. Allen expressed his creativity in his cello performances. I began to see how deciphering a biological system was comparable to figuring out a "harmony". I also enjoy both listening to and performing music and hope to strike a rewarding balance between personal and professional creativity as Dr. Allen did.

The two summers I spent at MBL had a profound effect on my approach to my studies and instilled in me a desire to learn as much as possible. Surrounded by distinguished scientists and taking advantage of daily lectures, I came to realize that learning is a privilege. My ability to grasp difficult concepts improved with my increased exposure to new fields.

During these summers of research, however, I realized how important human interactions are to me. In high school I spent two years helping my grandmother through the difficulties associated with age. After she died, I enjoyed helping the elderly at holiday dinners organized by our church. In losing my closest grandparent, I gained several hundred more. In grade school my father sustained multiple heart attacks and during my sophomore year he suffered a stroke. The following year was made more difficult when both my aunt and Dr. Allen developed cancer. During this period I began to see how illness and medicine related to the sciences I had been studying, and I realized this was the field I was most interested in pursuing.

I returned to Amherst determined to put my knowledge into my senior research project. In order to devote myself totally to this goal, I decided to wait a year before applying to medical school. My experience with and love of photography played a major role in our success as my aesthetic sense and desire to get good photographs of beautiful cells constantly led us to better pictures and an abundance of cytological information we had not expected.

While I have participated in research over the last four years, I have seen its applications help my own family. I would therefore gain satisfaction from involvement in both the research aspect of medicine and its practical applications in patient care.

Essay #43

My goal for wanting to attend medical school is not to become just another M.D. but instead to become a warm and caring physician who is willing and able to humbly serve the people and their community to bring about improvements for the present human condition. In order to accomplish such task one must have the necessary dedication, knowledge and love for others.

Dedication to a worthy goal is important because this is what enables one to accomplish things beyond the ordinary limit. In whatever one does, without dedication, he can only reach mediocrity. This summer, through the help of the U.C.C. (United Church of Christ), I had the opportunity to dedicate my vacation to working as a volunteer at a missionary hospital in a small town called Humacao in Puerto Rico. While working there I've gained practical experience in different departments of the hospital. The most learning experience was working as a physician's assistant at their Home Care Program. In this program, health care professionals commute for hours to reach isolated households in the countryside to give treatment to those poor patients who can not get to the hospital themselves. From working with these dedicated physicians I realized that a strong sense of dedication is the driving force that pushes one to achieve deeds that are beyond the limit of an ordinary doctor. That is why I want to become a humble, compassionate doctor who is sincerely dedicated to improving the human condition.

However, with dedication alone I can not accomplish this task; I need the necessary skills and knowledge which will enable me to take actions toward my goal. During my years at Cornell, I've concentrated on getting a well-rounded liberal education rather than a science-oriented premedical education. I've tried to study as many courses in humanities and social sciences as I could, and I'm also majoring in Spanish literature because I believe one must first be a well-rounded human being who can think before he can become a competent worker in any field of profession. Knowledge is not knowing a lot of scientific facts and data, but instead it's the ability to think creatively and analytically, the power of observation and problem solving, and the infinite curiosity to discover the unknown. This year I'll be doing undergraduate research on lipid biochemistry because I believe that exploring into what is unknown is equally important as mastering what is already known. I want to become a kind of a doctor who will expand the horizon of the current medical knowledge because the never-ending desire to understand the inexplicable is the key to the progress of the world.

Dedication and knowledge are indispensable elements in the making of a warm and caring physician; however, they are not sufficient. In order to become a "complete" doctor who is competent, compassionate and understanding, one must be able to love the mankind. In the future I want to become a loving doctor who has a warm, family-like relationship with each and every one of his patients, the kind of a doctor who can readily communicate and understand his patients on one-to-one basis because such doctor-patient communication is invaluable in treating a patient. During my undergraduate years I've been involved in a wide range of extracurricular and community activities from which I've learned a lot about human relations. I've also worked overseas where I've been exposed to different people and culture. From these experiences I've gained the patience, understanding and a caring heart, all of which are necessary in communcating and dealing with all kinds of difficult people and situation, and I believe this qualification will help me greatly in becoming a compassionate and understanding doctor who can readily meet the needs of the people.

Essay #44

My desire to become a physician originated during my childhood, a time when my father, who is himself a physician, served as my primary mentor and role model. As I matured, the initially blind longings he instilled in me were transformed into apprised aspirations and viable expectations. I have come to esteem medicine as a dynamic field promising a career filled with challenge and change. In addition, it offers the opportunity to have a positive impact on society while insuring a measure of respect and financial security. Equally appealing to me are medicine's clinical aspects, for I greatly value the chance to interact with a varying mix of people in diverse situations.

That these elements are indeed important career expectations for me has been self-substantiated by numerous personal experiences. Growing up in a family of seven, I have known all my life the pleasures of cooperation and interhuman relationships. In addition, my many years of participation in team sports have increased my proclivity for group interaction, as have my more recent experiences living with twenty other individuals in my fraternity house. This need for close contact and association with people has always been a prominent facet of my personality, and it is one I hope will find continued expression through clinical medicine.

I have also always felt the need to be challenged, and this has afforded me some very gratifying experiences. Entering college I had no prior exposure to secure myself a spot in the Crew program. This led to two very enjoyable seasons of rowing, and allowed me to develop some close friendships in addition to the techniques and skills of a new sport. Sportscasting was also foreign to me prior to college, but over the past three years I have managed to work my way up to the senior position among hockey commentators at the college radio station. This pursuit has not only proved to be exciting, but also quite beneficial as it has improved my extemporaneous oratory skills.

I have also tried to challenge myself academically at college, and this pledge bolstered my resolution to undertake study of the Chinese language. While these have perhaps been my most difficult courses, they have also been my most enjoyable. From them I have developed a fascination with the Chinese culture which not only has led me to major in this area, but, beginning this summer, I will undertake an intensive three month course of study in the People's Republic of China, followed by an additional three months of study in Taiwan. It is my hope that these next six months will not only afford me fluency in the Chinese language, but an intimate look at an alien culture and the opportunity to augment my intellectual and emotional growth, as well.

Though limited by space, it is my hope that these few preceeding examples demonstrate my commitment to the characteristics of a career in medicine. Furthermore, I have strengthened this commitment through extensive service as a hospital volunteer. Since high school I have worked at different hospitals in patient transport, intensive care, and pediatrics. My current volunteer work playing with hospitalized children typifies the whole range of these experiences. The immediate emotional gratification I receive from my work, though tempered by an often brutal reality, has made my attraction towards medicine even more genuine and concrete.

As I conclude, a Confucian aphorism comes to mind: "The wise embrace all knowledge, but they are most earnest about what is of the greatest importance." Throughout college I have been diligent in embracing many different streams of knowledge. However, graduation necessitates an estimation of these varied intellectual pursuits, and, for me, there is little question that, among them, my ambition to study medicine ranks supreme.

Essay #45

"If you don get paid, why the Hell do you work here?"
While working at the Pine Street Inn, Boston's largest
shelter for the homeless, this question came up often. Before
giving an honest answer, one is forced to do a lot of
soul searching. I could have, after all, chosen a more pleasant
placement than the Inn, where for ten hours a week I comforted and assisted hundreds of alcoholic and often deeply
disturbed individuals. These derelicts shared a misery too
profound for words.

In such an atmosphere of despair and frustration, one must
still try to find some achievement for your own piece of mind,
while dealing with a social system that has completely failed
these individuals. The Inn teaches you to strive for improvement no matter how small, and even though so much is needed. In trying your best at whatever you do, it is important to
understand your own limitations, both personal and within the
system. Several times I've spent hours talking to a "guest",
and have left the Inn beaming with a sense of accomplishment
only to be discouraged when a week later my new friend is on
the floor, quiet in unconsciousness except for an occasional
cough from lungs that only God could have designed to last
through such punishment. Compassion is born in places like
this, and can possess you totally if not kept in perspective.

A physician's practice in many ways parallels this experience.
His limitations are the scientific laws governing our bodies.
When fighting for another's life becomes your vocation, losing
to death becomes a hard pill to swallow. Our knowledge of
medicine is ever growing, yet the nemesis of death will always
be the final victor.

Why ride an emotional rollercoaster and volunteer at the
Pine Street Inn, or dedicate yourself to becoming a physician?
Because in helping people, you gain an understanding and
compassion that sensitizes you to a wide range of human
conditions, and makes you want to do your share in trying to
better them.

Essay #46

I was born in Hungary and received a well-rounded education complete with 10 years of extra-curricular piano, singing, ballet and language lessons. From an early age I was fascinated by the scientific and technological advances of the West to the extent that I decided to emigrate and, at the age of 12, began to study English in preparation for this move. I received a Ph.D. in Psychobiology from Eotvos Lorand University in Budapest in 1977 and left for the U.S.A. the same year.

I received a post-doctoral fellowship at the Neurology Department of the University of Pennsylvania Medical School. Here I learned about various brain imaging techniques such as Positron Emmission Tomography (PET), Nuclear Magnetic Resonance and regional Cerebral Blood Flow and developed a strong interest in functional neuroanatomy. I devised a PET study which demonstrated an asymmetry of glucose metabolism in the human posterior parietal lobes during the performance of directed attentional tasks. Furthermore, I demonstrated an asymmetry of cortical control of heart rate in humans under conditions of unilateral barbituration of the hemispheres. Neither of the above had been previously reported in the literature. I was also involved in projects studying the impact of cognitive tasks on cerebral glucose metabolism, glucose metabolism changes in epilepsy and in schizophrenia.

In 1982 I was invited to present my findings at Behavioral Neurology Grand Rounds at Beth Israel Hospital of Harvard Medical School and was offered a 2 year NIH institutional National Research Service Award. At Harvard I worked on a study describing the distribution of acetylocholinesteraze in the primate cortex and a study describing the cortico-cortical connectivity of the temporal poles of primates. I also had the opportunity to attend Neurology Grand Rounds and Behavioural Neurology Grand Rounds on a weekly basis for 2 years. This experience was my first exposure to brain lesioned patients and it made me realize that clinical observation is perhaps the richest source of information in the study of neuroanatomical correlates of human behaviour. I found the clinical experience intellectually fascinating as well as emotionally stimulating and it triggered a strong desire in me to become a physician.

Two years ago I enrolled in the post-baccalaureate pre-medical program of Hunter College. Last year I had the singular honour of being placed at the top of the list of accepted candidates at both the Cornell and Mount Sinai Medical School linkage programs. I have chosen the Cornell program due to its newly established PET facility as well as its exceptional reputation in the neurosciences.

Essay #47

Before coming to Brandeis, my decision to pursue a medical career was based solely on my interest in the sciences. However, my experiences over the past three years have been very self revealing, and not only has my reasoning for pursuing a medical career been modified, but also the type of career which I plan to pursue.

My extracurricular and work experience at Brandeis have helped me to realize both my desire to interact and work with others and my skill and ability to do so. As captain of both intramural football and basketball teams, I voluntarily placed upon myself an added responsibility. While this responsibility was at times a slight burden, I found that being captain made the overall experience more challenging and exciting. Working at Brandeis for the past two years as a chemistry group tutor has also enabled me to interact with and instruct others. Occasionally this became a humbling experience after struggling with a problem or concept with which I was not familiar. However, the gratitude expressed by the students, and my own ability to grapple with the problems, almost always made it rewarding and worthwhile.

In addition to my work at Brandeis, I spent the past two summers working at The Rockefeller University in Manhattan in a biochemistry lab. Last summer I was given an independent research project involving the determination of the metabolism of a certain super androgen. I found it to be a fascinating educational experience, and I learned firsthand the manner in which biomedical research is done and the many frustrations and obstacles which inherently go along with it. My summer work has been very inspirational. This summer I will begin my senior honors research in biochemistry for which I was awarded the Doris Brewer Cohen Award. I now plan on doing research as part of my career. However, working in the lab has also made me realize that I do not want to do research exclusively. At times I felt somewhat isolated, and I believe that I would be better suited in a career which would integrate research and application of my scientific knowledge to real life situations.

My decision to pursue a medical career now has a much more solid foundation upon which to build. I believe that my desires and talents will be best fulfilled and utilized in a medical career which involves both research and clinical work.

Essay #48

Several incidents, over the past five years, have been major influences on my decision to become a physician.

I recall performing an emergency test on a boy suspected of having appendicitis. The next morning I encountered his mother, and was struck by the look of concern on her face. This made me realize the importance of the contribution I had made to the attempt to save the boy's life.

Even though I found working as a technician gratifying, an event occured that made me want to participate more meaningfully in the care of patients. While working in a medically underserved area, I performed a test for bleeding and clotting time on a man with a snake-bite. The patient died because of the unavailability of a doctor. Watching the dead man I felt a strong sense of inadequacy because, even though I had known the test results were abnormal, I could do nothing to help the patient. I decided to pursue a career that would enable me to make a greater contribution to the care of patients.

One experience as a resesarch aide gave me some appreciation of how doctors might feel when faced with a frustrating situation, and how they might deal with such a situation. After working on a synthesis of a labelled amino acid for several weeks, I isolated a product that was totally unexpected. I felt frustrated and defeated. After careful examination I discovered that the reaction mechanism was different from the one proposed. I had actually discovered the true reaction mechanism. This experience taught me that regardless of your hard work and dedication, there will always be instance of failure, and the best way to deal with these failures is to use them as learning experiences.

Three aspects of my character that I consider important are my self-discipline, my ability to relate to others, and my honesty. Honesty to myself is of special importance because it enables me to identify my strengths and weaknesses, and to be aware of my limitations.

I am confident that I will be able to function well as a physician because of my character, and the experience I have acquired. I have been exposed to various aspects of health care, and I am comfortable working in a hospital environment. Having worked on call I have learned to deal with the stress of making crucial decisions quickly and working long hours with little or no sleep. Thus, I can begin to appreciate the demands a career in medicine will make on me. However, I know it is what I want, and I am willing to work hard to succeed.

Essay #49

I worked in the observatory this summer as a computer programmer. Working in programming was a valuable learning experience but even more valuable was observing the interaction
between people in the maintenance staff, the technical staff,
and the scientific staff. It was often interesting to see how important was all their work to keep the observatory running
smoothly. I will relate what I observed during one of my days
of work.

This day was very important for one of the scientists. After
about five to six years of planning an experiment, the day for
performing the experiment had arrived. The experiment was
done in conjunction with the Space Shuttle. At about midnight
the Shuttle would boost its engines right above the radio-telescope;
gasses from the engines would disturb the ionosphere making a
hole in it. This disturbance would be observed from the tele-
scope for about twelve hours.

By 11:00 pm the experimenter had all the equipment ready to
observe the hole. The only missing information was the exact
coordinates at which the Shuttle would burn the ionosphere
and this information would be given in a phone call from
Houston at about 11:45 pm.

At about 11:30 pm a technician reparing a phone line damaged
by a thunderstorm accidentally turned on a switch that caused
a shutdown of all phone communications. The closest phone to the
observatory is about half an hour away by car. The atmosphere
in the observatory was tense. Some other workers were teasing
the technician while he tried to recover the communication
lines. They were telling him that due to his blunder the experiment would fail. The experimenter was nervous; the technician
was even more nervous.

Sometime around 11:50 p.m. the technician fixed the line,
communication with Houston was possible, and the experimenter
received the coordinates. The data was collected and everything
looked as if it was all right.

I realized afterwards that nothing of what I related here will
be known to someone looking at a research paper on this experiment. A lot of the work done by the maintenance employees,
the technicians, and the scientists remains hidden and unrecognized by someone just looking at the results. But all this work

is important and essential to the progress of research.

Also unnoticed remain the human qualities of all these personnel, which in a given circumstance may affect the outcome of their joint endeavor. In my example, the worker's response of enjoying the technician's misfortune could have impaired his ability to fix the line quickly. In other instances workers were extremely helpful to one another, and better than usual working situations were created. Whenever human beings interact, human qualities will show up, some favorable and some unfavorable, and in the same way that they could affect the result of an experiment they could also have an effect in other fields of work.

Essay# 50

During my secondary education at The Hill School, in Pottstown, Pennsylvania, I organized a voluntary program to assist the mentally retarded, especially those ignored by their families. Most were middle-aged men suffering from loneliness or depression, and many were given to self-inflicted violence. By arranging surprise parties and picnics, or teaching them songs and games, we gave them companionship and strove to remove their desolation and depression. I have often wondered about the lives of my friends at The Pennhurst House, where they resided. Although I was happy to be able to lead them to see their lives positively through the daily activities we offered, I felt that I was not doing anything really to help cure them. My understanding of their unspoken sufferings made me want to be in a position where I could alleviate the pain in their lives.

My experiences at the Cornell University Medical College reinforced my decision to become a physician. I spent one semester in the Cornell Field Study Program and three summers at the medical college in order to learn about both academic and clinical aspects of medicine. On weekdays, I worked in a cardio-electrophysiology laboratory, using sodium-selective and calcium-selective microelectrodes in order to investigate pharmacological aspects of Digitalis on intracellular sodium and calcium ion activities in cardiac Purkinje fibers. I worked with little supervision and learned to be creative and patient in carrying out the projects. The intellectual challenge and satisfaction that I received, especially after achieving progress, made me seriously consider continuing this learning experience. On weekends, I worked as a volunteer in the emergency room, carrying blood and body fluid samples to the pathology department and transferring emergency patients to their designated rooms. My hospital experiences confirmed my beliefs about what a physician should be in a hospital: As an investigator of diseases, a physician must be competent in his field of medicine; furthermore, as a leader of a healing team, he must know how to lead a group and to communicate well with his fellow workers; but, most importantly, as a counselor, he must be compassionate towards his patients and be willing to guide them. Medicine requires competency, communication, and compassion. Reflecting on the experiences that I had both at the medical research laboratory and the emergency room, I found that I liked what I would do as a physician, not only to fulfill my daily responsibilities, but also to take up the challenges of solving new and crucial problems in patient care and medical research.

My undergraduate years have challenged and improved my intellectual creativity, social responsiblity, and personal integrity. Taking the intitiative to design an independent research course and a Field Study Program for a semester, I gained much perspective about the nature of scientific studies. Fulfilling responsibility as a student representative in the University Board on Health Service, and in the AIDS Prevention Committee, I learned to educate the community about the importance of preventive attitude towards health. As a tutor in the Mathematics Department in the College of Arts and Sciences, and as an orientation counselor, I enjoyed the role of a teacher and learned to be a more effective communicator. As captain of an intramural soccer team and as a Junior Varsity Squash player, I developed not only stamina, but also self-discipline and organizational skills. Taking photography, playing the piano, and travelling across various cultures, I have broadened myself and gained much understanding about the global world and the people.

I appreciate the variety of experiences I have had, not only because they have prepared me for the diversity I expect to encounter in a medical career, but also because they taught me how to lead my life; to use my potential for those who need the medical help. I would like to pursue both clinical and academic medicine. Each will enrich the other in improving patient care and medical knowledge. I know that the M.D. degree will not automatically guarantee my becoming a good physician; self-education throughout my life is essential. Believing, like Dr. Bernard Lown, that "those who can see the invisible can do the impossible," I look forward to using my Cornell University liberal arts and sciences education as a solid basis for acquiring the further training necessary to become a competent and caring physician.

Epilogue

Destiny is not a matter of chance, it's a matter of choice. It's not something to be waited for, it's something to be achieved. Robert Browning

Medicine is not only an applied science, it is also an art, and the art of medicine lies in the healer's insight, empathy, and ability to communicate with the patient effectively. Young physicians must enter medicine compassionate and dedicated to their professional calling.

We stress these essential qualities because, all too often, applicants who could be great physicians get discouraged from applying. If you have a sincere interest is serving the sick, **don't underestimate your fitness for medicine.** A low grade point average or mediocre MCAT score should not dissuade you from becoming a physician.

Follow the formula we have outlined, have a positive outlook toward medicine and the admissions process, persevere, and you *will* be offered an acceptance to medical school. Do your best—no one can ask for more. Remember, top-notch applicants with the proper outlook and personality are always in high demand.

The bureaucracy and stress involved in the admissions process may cloud your original goal and diminish your desire. Try not to let yourself be disillusioned and discouraged, and be patient. In time, you *will* be practicing medicine, and you *will* be in a position to really help others.

We still recall vividly the hassle of marketing ourselves and the anxiety we felt during the admission process. Writing the essay, completing applications on time, buying an appropriate suit to project the proper image, sweating during the interview, checking the mailbox several times a day for an acceptance/rejection letter—it's all just part of the rites of passage to medicine. Repeatedly, we would ask, "Is it *really* worth it?"

Well, now we can honestly answer, "Yes." There is always something new to learn about disease, patients, and even yourself. Medicine becomes a philosophy that assigns meaning and purpose to our society. Most significantly, there is no greater feeling than knowing that every day as a doctor you are able to make a difference in the life of another.

We wish you the best of luck in your career. You have made it this far, and taking the initiative to read this book shows you are heading in the right direction. Have confidence in yourself and your accomplishments, and one day you *will* become a physician!

About the Authors

John A. Zebala is an M.D.-Ph.D. candidate at Cornell University Medical College in New York City. He received his B.S. in Biomedical Engineering from the University of Southern California. He hopes to apply modern principles of molecular biology to solve basic clinical problems.

Daniel B. Jones recently graduated from Cornell University Medical College and is now a resident at Barnes Hospital in St. Louis. He graduated with an A.B. in Biology & Society from Cornell University. He is currently a member of the American Medical Association, and he plans a career in general surgery.

Stephanie Brickner Jones recently graduated from Washington University School of Medicine after completing her first two years of medical school at New York University School of Medicine. She received a B.S. in Biochemistry with Honors and Distinction from Cornell University. She will begin her residency training in anesthesiology at Barnes Hospital after an internship in internal medicine at the Jewish Hospital of St. Louis.

More Great Books
from Mustang Publishing

Working in T.V. News: The Insider's Guide by Carl Filoretto, with Lynn Setzer. Written by veteran television journalists, this is the most practical and most thorough guide to the T.V. news business available. With complete information on the variety of jobs in a T.V. news department, the hard truth about salaries and hours, advice on the perfect résumé tape, a description of an average day in a T.V. news operation, and much more, this book is a must for anyone considering a career in broadcast journalism. *Available November, 1992.* **$10.95**

The One Hour College Applicant by Lois Rochester & Judy Mandell. Let's face it: applying to college is not brain surgery! There's no reason to read an 8,000-page book before your fill out a college application. However, applicants *do* need to be informed and organized before they apply, and this book tells you everything you need to know—from tips on choosing the right college to ideas on writing a great essay—in easy-to-read, outline form. It's the only application guide most students will ever need—or want. *"It simplifies the whole process and alleviates the stress."* —Kliatt Young Adult Book Guide. **$8.95**

The Complete Book of Beer Drinking Games by Griscom, Rand, & Johnston. With over 400,000 copies sold, this book is without a doubt the imbiber's bible! From descriptions of classic beer games like Quarters and Blow Pong to hilarious new contests like Slush Fund and Beer Hunter—plus lots of funny cartoons, essays, and lists—this book remains the party essential. *"The 'Animal House' of literature."* —Dallas Morning News. **$6.95**

Let's Blow thru Europe by Neenan & Hancock. The ultimate guide for the "15-cities-in-14-days" traveler, this is the funniest, most irreverent, and definitely most honest travel guide ever written. With this book, you can blow off the boring museums and minor cathedrals and instead find the great bars, restaurants, and fun stuff in all the major cities of Europe. *"A riot!"* —The Daily Northwestern (Northwestern U.). **$10.95**

Festival Europe! Fairs & Celebrations throughout Europe by Margaret M. Johnson. What's the best—and least expensive—way to interact with Europeans and their cultures? Attend their myriad festivals, celebrations, fairs, and parades, most of which are free!

From the somber Holy Blood Procession in Bruges to the wild Oktoberfest in Munich, this guide will help any traveler have a terrific, festive time in Europe. *"An excellent book for the serious traveler."* —Bookviews. **$10.95**

Europe on 10 Salads a Day by Mary Jane & Greg Edwards. A must for the health-conscious traveler! From gourmet Indian cuisine in Spain to terrific take-out pizza in Italy, this book describes over 200 health food/vegetarian restaurants throughout Europe. *"Don't go to Europe without it"* —Vegetarian Times. **$9.95**

Europe for Free by Brian Butler. If you're on a tight budget—or if you just love a bargain—this is the book for you! With descriptions of thousands of things to do and see for free all over Europe, you'll save lots of lira, francs, and pfennigs. *"Well-organized and packed with ideas"* —Modern Maturity. **$8.95**

Also in this series:
London for Free by Brian Butler. **$7.95**
DC for Free by Brian Butler. **$6.95**
Hawaii for Free by Frances Carter. **$6.95**

The Nepal Trekker's Handbook by Amy R. Kaplan. This book guides trekkers through every aspect of planning and enjoying a trek through Nepal—one of the world's most magnificent adventures. From medical advice to cultural *faux-pas*, it's an essential guide. *"A must"* — Midwest Book Review. **$9.95**

Australia: Where the Fun Is by Goodyear & Skinner. From the best pubs in Sydney to the cheapest motels in Darwin to the greatest hikes in Tasmania, this guide by two recent Yale grads details all the fun stuff Down Under—on and off the beaten path. *"Indispensable"* — Library Journal. **$12.95**

Mustang books should be available at your local bookstore. If not, send a check or money order for the price of the book, plus $1.50 postage per book, to Mustang Publishing, P.O. Box 3004, Memphis, TN 38173 U.S.A.

Allow three weeks for delivery. For rush, one-week delivery, add $3.00 to the total. *International orders*: Please pay in U.S. funds, and add $5.00 to the total for Air Mail.

For a complete catalog of Mustang books, send $1.00 and a stamped, self-addressed, business size envelope to Catalog Request, Mustang Publishing, P.O. Box 3004, Memphis, TN 38173.